# The 3 Phases of Lyme

## Conners Clinic Clear Lyme Protocols

DR KEVIN CONNERS

Fellowship in Integrative Cancer Therapy

Fellowship in Anti-Aging, Regenerative, and Functional Medicine

American Academy of Anti-Aging Medicine

*The 3 Phases of Lyme*
Conners Clinic Clear Lyme Protocols

Copyright © 2016, 2020 by Dr. Kevin Conners

*Published by*
Conners Clinic
ConnersClinic.com

# CONTENTS

# FOREWORD

Many doctors speak on disease from the third-person perspective, saying things like "In my experience with Lyme Disease patients, they should…" While this is understandable and comes from people who are trying their best to help others that are ill, there is undoubtedly a big difference when a doctor has personal experience with the disease you suffer from.

I personally struggled with Chronic Lyme Disease for many years. In fact, Lyme Disease nearly killed me! There were days where I'd close my eyes at night and not think I'd make it to the next day. I was so sick I spent most days in bed, unable to take care of my young children, let alone myself.

Yet I never gave up. I knew God had plans for my life beyond being sick with Lyme. I gradually made my way back to health, slowly gaining ground as I learned from other patients and great doctors. One of those great doctors was my friend and mentor, Dr. Kevin Conners. He has committed his life to others and I still thank God every day for him and all that he did for me.

I met Dr. Conners in 2013 when I was better but still struggling with my recovery. He taught me new concepts that helped me gain my life back. In fact, his care and guidance catapulted my healing so much so that my husband and I welcomed our third child in 2016! My body had made a full recovery and to this day I still use the concepts he shares in this book to keep myself and the people in my care healthy.

Dr. Conners' life-changing concepts will probably be new to many of you as they were to me in the beginning. Some readers will definitely have that *Ah-ha* moment where they realize what they've been doing wrong and how they can fix it.

Understanding Autoimmune Lyme was a new concept to me and has made all the difference in my recovery. I had been helping my body destroy itself. I personally helped Dr. Conners with his new formulations of supplements for each of the 3 phases of Lyme and was as excited as he when they came out.

I'm sure you'll agree that the simple yet profound information in this book will change the way you treat Lyme patients if you are a practitioner or help direct your own care if you are a patient. Though you may need to read this book over several times to truly digest the content and put it into action, it has the potential to change your life. It changed mine and I am forever grateful.

In your service,
Dr. Kelly Halderman

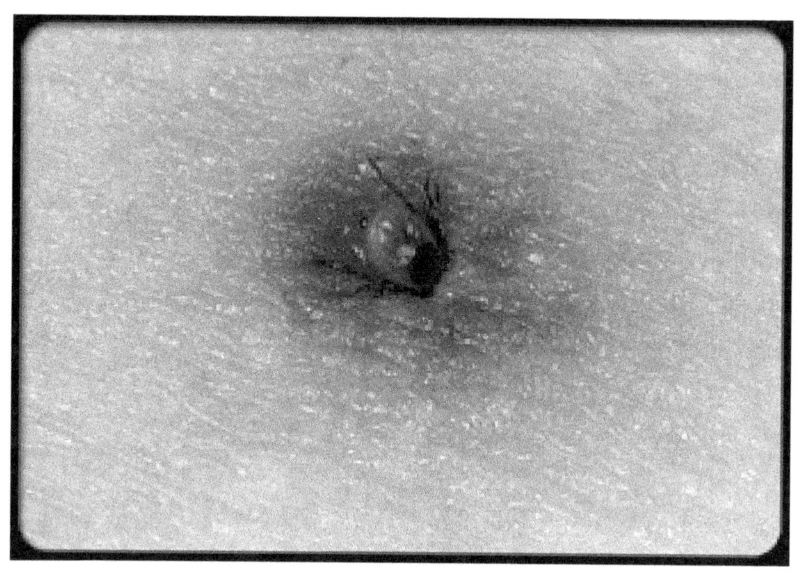

# PREFACE

Let me begin by stating that this book is an updated and refined version of my first book on Lyme with added protocols to help those that I may never be able to see. As I stated in the foreword of my first book on Lyme Disease, I've had Lyme three times now. Honestly, I'll most likely have it again since, at the time of this writing, my wife and I live on a small hobby farm where my best stress-reliever seems to be spending hours on my zero-turn mower listening to books through my noise-cancelling headphones. Let's just say that I am exposed to a **lot** of ticks.

If you've read my first book you've heard me tell my story of how we once lived in the middle of the 280-acre woods. Like Pooh and piglet survived *off-grid* and though our home was slightly better than a hollowed tree, we grew most of our own food and had to pump our water by hand. Sparing you from all of the details, God was preparing us for our next phase of life – full-time missionary work in Mexico.

I'll spare you the details of my past because, quite frankly, that's not why you are reading this book. However, I will share with you the *life phrase* the has shaped my decisions for the past several decades:

## "If you are claiming to be a person of FAITH,
## Then live a life that requires faith!"

More on this later, but for now let's just say that whatever struggles you currently find yourself in, whether it's drowning in brain fog, exhausted in pain, or emotionally spent, this book is going to challenge you, and that is my goal.

Disclaimer: I cannot take credit for what's in this book. The Book of Ecclesiastes states, "What has been will be again, what has been done will be done again; there is nothing new under the sun." (Ecc 1:9) Information contained here is simply a small piece of 28 years of practical experience learning from

4

other doctors who've paved the way, scientists dedicated to finding answers, and patients who share their stories. This is in no way a complete work; it is a start. I am not an Infectious Disease Specialist, I am a chiropractor with advanced training in neurology, integrative cancer, anti-aging and functional medicine, nutrition, etc. I am simply attempting to convey information and opinion; this is not a substitute for medical care. Any and all information in this book is NOT a substitute for standard medical care. Please consult your physician before considering any information in this book. This book is an opinion, not a protocol, it is the reader's responsibility to seek appropriate medical care and to understand that this book does not suggest or imply that treating Lyme Disease is anything but reserved for appropriate medical establishments. Please see the full disclaimer at the end of this book.

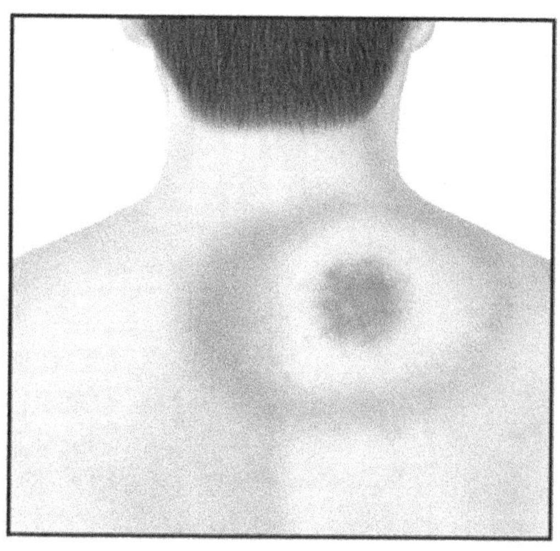

# REDEFINING A
# MISUNDERSTOOD DISEASE

*"~~Russia~~ (Lyme) is a riddle wrapped in a mystery inside an enigma."*
*Winston Churchill*

## What Is It?

To most in the medical community, Lyme Disease is an enigma. To those suffering with it, it is a riddle. There still remains an argument in traditional medicine whether Chronic Lyme even exists. The general stance by many state medical boards is that it should not be treated with antibiotic therapy until a positive titer is found at which time the patient has often progressed beyond antibiotic help.

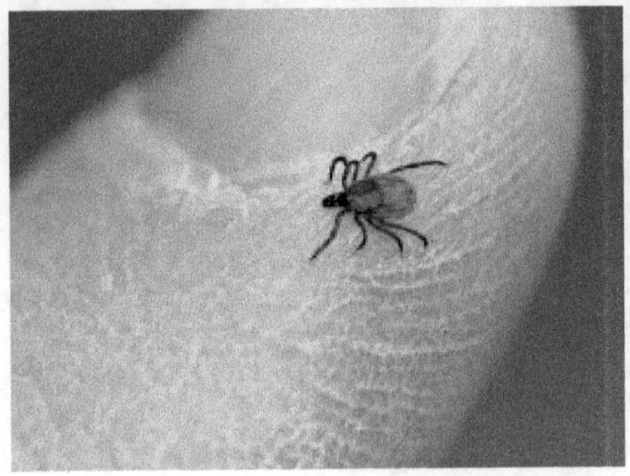

This observed ineffectiveness of antibiotic therapy leads doctors that are unfamiliar with the 3 phases of Lyme to assume the patient is crazy. People are told to seek psychiatric help, put on antidepressants, and have been made to feel like they are hypochondriacs. I hear stories like this every day!

But we know differently! Chronic Lyme Disease is a seriously complex, multi-system, inflammatory, autoimmune disease that is triggered by the bacterial lipoproteins (lipopolysaccharides) produced by the spiral-shaped bacteria of the family called Borrelia. Though most doctors may acknowledge Acute Lyme, as you cannot continue to ignore the evidence of an identifiable bacterial infection, the inability of antibiotics to kill it after a period of time is what is in question.

This is what this book is all about.

8

# Borrelia – The Italian Mob Taking Over Your Cells

The problem with the Borrelia family of parasites (currently over 90 by count including all the co-infections that tend to tag along with those having Lyme) is that they are difficult to detect, isolate, grow, and study in the laboratory. This means that our technical knowledge of this pathogen is poor and misunderstood. The disease can affect every tissue and every major organ system in the body. Clinically, it can appear as a chronic arthralgia (joint pain), fibromyalgia (fibrous connective tissue and muscle pain), chronic fatigue (affecting the brain and glands), immune dysfunction, and as neurological disease. Lyme may even be fatal in severe cases depending on severity and the organ being attacked.

The diagnosis of Lyme Disease *should be* primarily based upon clinical evidence, but time and time again I see patients who are unable to receive necessary, immediate antibiotics until labs are run. This is a HUGE mistake! There are currently no perfect laboratory tests that are definitive for Lyme Disease (though I will discuss my recommendations later).

Without arguing test accuracy, the time delay of blood draw to result is the real problem. Even if all Lyme tests were flawless, non-treatment for even a few hours can lead to progression into the second phase of Lyme, where the desired Phase One treatment (antibiotics) will now prove relatively ineffective.

Borrelia is a family of bacteria, not a Chicago mob. Though sufferers may argue the latter. Lyme is quickly becoming one of the fastest growing (spreading) infectious diseases. At the time of this writing, we are getting calls and emails from people around the world with symptoms local doctors are unable to diagnose. The bulls-eye skin rash that commonly develops following the bite of an infected tick is often absent. The disease can begin with flu-like symptoms but more often than not, patients either do not experience early symptoms or fail to remember the initial incident that is now causing their chronic, debilitating, and often misdiagnosed disorder.

I wrote this book as an extra and urgent warning for everyone. Acute Lyme Disease (Phase 1), left untreated, most often will progress to Phase 2 (Chronic Lyme), then Phase 3 (Autoimmune Lyme), which is devastating the lives of hundreds of thousands of individuals (most never suspecting Lyme as the cause of their disease), and we are all at risk. Most are misdiagnosed and mistreated. In many cases of Lyme Disease, a correct diagnosis doesn't occur until after several months or more often many years of suffering with the disease. Even if the blood tests were perfect, waiting a week for the results may be too late! By then it may have caused severe illness, disability, or permanent damage. The disease is widespread, and the prevalence is significantly higher than reported by health officials.

There are some key factors that exist in the medical community regarding Lyme Disease; they go a long way in explaining why Chronic Lyme is often misdiagnosed and mistreated. However, possibly the greatest reason that Acute Lyme (Phase 1) becomes Chronic Lyme Disease (Phase 2 and then 3) is the following criteria (hoops) that standard medical doctors must jump through to legally diagnose:

*"Internationally recognized criteria for the diagnosis of Lyme borreliosis are based upon stringent interpretation of serological tests for specific antibodies to B. burgdorferi sensu lato. The criteria recommended in the USA (from the Centers for Disease Control and Prevention), Europe (i.e. MiQ 20-00 Germany) and the UK are:*
*• Serum samples for the detection of antibodies to B. burgdorferi should be analyzed by a two-test procedure:*
> *- A sensitive screening test (e.g. ELISA or IFA). All samples judged to be reactive or equivocal in the screening test should then be confirmed by*
> *- A Western blot for antibodies to specific B. burgdorferi antigens. The Western blot should only be used in succession with an ELISA or IFA test. Detailed interpretive criteria for Western blots differ between Europe and the USA, to take into account differences in the geographic distribution of the infecting genospecies.*

The evidence continues to mount that Chronic Lyme Disease exists and must be addressed by the medical community if solutions are to be found[2]. 34% of a "population-based, retrospective cohort study in Massachusetts" were found to have arthritis or recurrent arthralgias, neurocognitive impairment, and neuropathy or myelopathy, a mean of 6 years after treatment for Lyme Disease (LD)[3]. 62% of "a cohort of 215 consecutively treated LD patients in Westchester County" were found to have arthralgias, arthritis, and cardiac or neurologic involvement with or without fatigue a mean of 3.2 years after treatment.[4]

---

[1] "Unorthodox and Unvalidated Laboratory Tests in the Diagnosis of Lyme Borreliosis and in Relation to Medically Unexplained Symptom", Duerden, B.I., UK Health Protection Agency Official Report on Lyme Disease

[2] Proof That Chronic Lyme Disease Exists, Daniel J. Cameron, Department of Medicine, Northern Westchester Hospital, Mt. Kisco, NY 10549, USA, Received 11 December 2009; Accepted 26 March 2010

[3] N. A. Shadick, C. B. Phillips, E. L. Logigian, et al., "The long-term clinical outcomes of Lyme Disease. A population-based retrospective cohort study," Annals of Internal Medicine, vol. 121, no. 8, pp. 560–567, 1994

[4] E. S. Asch, D. I. Bujak, M. Weiss, M. G. E. Peterson, and A. Weinstein, "Lyme Disease: an infectious and postinfectious syndrome," Journal of Rheumatology, vol. 21, no. 3, pp. 454–461, 1994

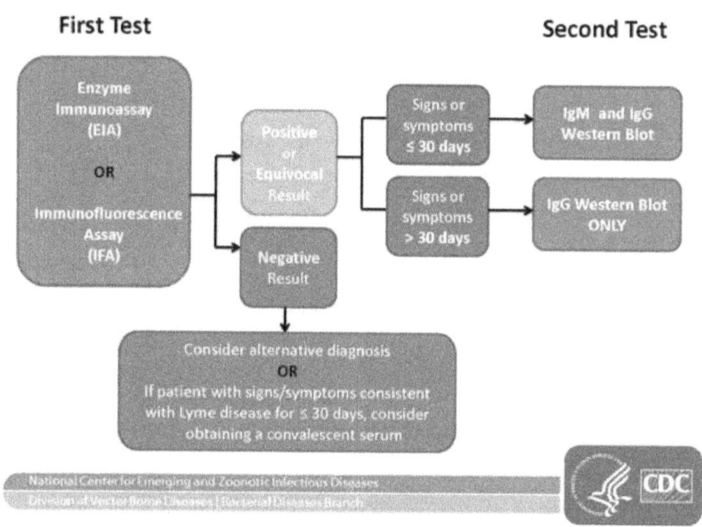



According to Cameron, "There is no objective way to rule out an active infection. Lab tests that can be very helpful in confirming a clinical diagnosis of Lyme Disease (such as the ELISA and Western blot tests) are not useful in determining whether the infection has been adequately treated.

Common LD symptoms such as Bell's palsy, erythema migrans rash, meningitis, arthritis, or heart block, which are included in the current surveillance definitions, can be useful in *ruling in* Lyme Disease, but the absence or disappearance of these symptoms cannot *rule out* an ongoing infection.

A population-based, retrospective cohort study of individuals with a history of LD revealed that they were significantly more likely to have joint pain, memory impairment, and poor functional status due to pain than persons without a history of LD, even though there were no signs of objective findings on physical examination or neurocognitive testing[5]. Two recent mouse studies revealed that spirochetes persist despite antibiotic therapy and that standard diagnostic tests are not able to detect their presence.[6] [7] In sum, there are no clinical or laboratory markers that identify the eradication of the pathogen.


Let us begin.

[5] N. A. Shadick, C. B. Phillips, O. Sangha, et al., "Musculoskeletal and neurologic outcomes in patients with previously treated Lyme Disease," Annals of Internal Medicine, vol. 131, no. 12, pp. 919–926, 1999

[6] E. Hodzic, S. Feng, K. Holden, K. J. Freet, and S. W. Barthold, "Persistence of Borrelia burgdorferi following antibiotic treatment in mice," Antimicrobial Agents and Chemotherapy, vol. 52, no. 5, pp. 1728–1736, 2008. View at Publisher · View at Google Scholar · View at PubMed

[7] H. Yrjänäinen, J. Hytönen, K.-O. Söderström, J. Oksi, K. Hartiala, and M. K. Viljanen, "Persistent joint swelling and borrelia-specific antibodies in Borrelia garinii-infected mice after eradication of vegetative spirochetes with antibiotic treatment," Microbes and Infection, vol. 8, no. 8, pp. 2044–2051, 2006

# My Definition of Lyme Disease Progression – The Three Phases of Lyme

## Phase 1: Acute Infection

In Phase 1, the patient **still** has the ability to **kill** the disease with an antibiotic. This is why I **highly** recommend that those living in Lyme-infested areas have antibiotics on hand to use should they develop symptoms in Lyme season. This is **only** open for a **window** of time, i.e. once you move into Phase 2, the ability to completely kill Lyme with antibiotic therapy is greatly reduced!

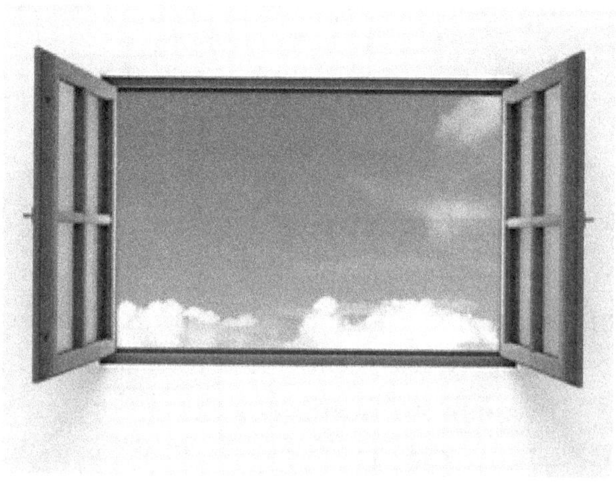

*The* window of opportunity *to* kill *Lyme in the Acute Phase can be very short.*

15

## Phase 2: Chronic Lyme

Chronic Lyme, Phase 2, begins the moment the first bacterium **exit** the bloodstream and **enter** the intracellular space (go inside the cell and hide). This phase still may be treated with antibiotics and immune-boosting nutraceuticals **but** it will be a **long**, drawn-out treatment plan and, in the case of long-term antibiotic use, there will be considerable damage to the gut and other cell membranes. Though it is better than Phase 3, this phase is still horrible and has left many devastated.

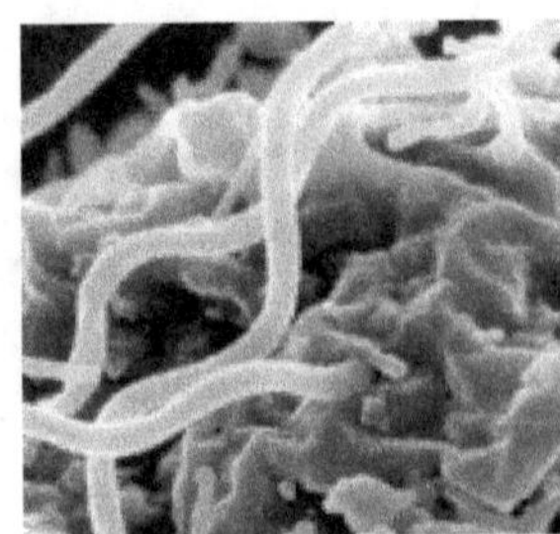

*A scanning electron microscope image of Borrelia burgdorferi penetrating a human B cell (in vitro), at a magnification of approximately 89,000.*
Photo Credit: David W. Dorward, Ph.D.
NIH Rocky Mountain Labs, MT.

## Phase 3: Autoimmune Lyme

When the patient's condition continues to linger, the immune system is constantly trying to kill it – this is normal. However, in doing so, the *killer* side of the immune system, the Th1 response, fires to kill the pathogen and is unable to enter the cell to destroy those bacteria that have entered. This will eventually calm the Th1 response and set-off a B-cell (Th2) immune response in an attempt to find the bacteria (the antigen) and make antibodies against the bug, thereby *tagging* the bacteria (with the antibody) allowing quick detection and destruction.

As this Th1–Th2 response cycles over time and the B cells continue to be unable to create antibodies to the specific antigen (due to the bacteria's ability to hide inside the cell), the immune system may begin to make antibodies against the cells themselves. ***This*** is what an autoimmune disease is and exactly how ***every*** autoimmune disorder begins! THIS phase (Phase 3, Autoimmune) is really what this book is all about! These patients are miserable, and it is the autoimmune phase of Lyme that is deadly.

See the videos on our website to help clarify at
**ConnersClinic.com/lyme**

## Why is Lyme so Frequently Misdiagnosed?

I don't believe that it is just my office that attracts people who have had physicians frequently overlook cases of Lyme Disease simply because they don't know the complex pathogenesis of the disease. Nearly every week I hear someone telling me a story of how they believed they had an Acute Lyme attack, had evidence of a tick bite and experienced typical symptoms suggesting Lyme, only to engage in an argument with their primary doctor and leave untreated.

Lyme Disease may cause well over 100 different symptoms; the common arthralgia (joint pain) is one symptom that most physicians are familiar with; however, it is only one of many symptoms caused by Lyme Disease.

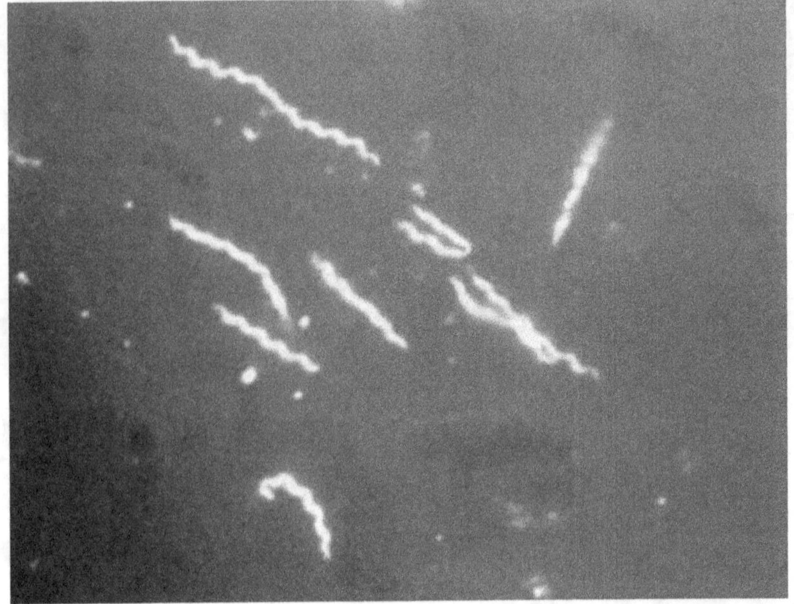

CLD Spirochetes

"The evidence continues to mount that Chronic Lyme Disease exists and must be addressed by the medical community if solutions are to be found. Four National Institutes of Health (NIH) trials validated the existence and severity of late stage Lyme. Despite the evidence, there are physicians

18

who continue to deny its existence and severity, which can hinder efforts to find a solution."[8]

Understand that you can get Lyme Disease multiple times. I am a perfect example; I had and cured Phase 1 Lyme Disease years ago and then was re-infected by a new, Acute Lyme bite. In a study that revealed Lyme can be killed with antibiotics if caught in the *bacterial phase*, the author states, "Our data provide compelling evidence that courses of antibiotics that are recommended by Infectious Disease Society of America regularly cure early Lyme Disease," said Nadelman, a professor of medicine in the division of infectious diseases at New York Medical College in Valhalla, in a telephone interview. "When people have early Lyme Disease again, it's likely due to a new infection due to a new tick bite."[9]

Most doctors don't know that laboratory tests are often useless and misleading – some reports suggest a 60-70% false negative rate! The laboratory isolation and identification of Borrelia is rarely successful; and no clinical test currently exists that can definitively diagnose Lyme Disease with 100% accuracy. This is why a diagnosis of Lyme Disease should be heavily based upon clinical information such as history, symptoms, and response to therapy.

---

[8] Interdiscip Perspect Infect Dis. 2010;2010:876450. doi: 10.1155/2010/876450. Epub 2010 May 25., Proof that Chronic Lyme Disease exists. Cameron DJ. Source: Department of Medicine, Northern Westchester Hospital, Mt. Kisco, NY 10549, USA

[9] Chronic Lyme Disease Discounted as New Infections Blamed By Michelle Fay Cortez - Nov 14, 2012 11:00 PM CT

There is an art to medicine when dealing with Lyme Disease and experienced physicians must use keen clinical skills and judgment as well as cutting edge diagnostic techniques such as Applied Kinesiology, FCT therapy, and down-home clinical experience when dealing with suspect Lyme Disease patients.

I liken modern medicine to auto mechanics. There was a time when an astute mechanic could listen to an engine and declare that the first lifter was sticking. Now we have become so sophisticated that without a $20,000 computer it is nearly impossible to accurately diagnose a car's problem. Though mechanics may have retained much of their working knowledge, it appears that most physicians have not. They seem lost without an MRI, CT scan, and lab work. I am not saying that there isn't great information derived from such advanced tools, but good old-fashioned diagnostic skills can become forgotten. Therefore, clinical diagnosis (and the competence to do so) should be made based on the physician's knowledge of the disease.[10]

If a physician is going to rely solely on laboratory tests to confirm a diagnosis of Lyme, they will be wrong more often than not! Most MDs don't know that Borrelia produce a large variety of toxic bacterial lipoproteins and they aren't familiar with the way these lipopolysaccharides cause the

---

[10] "The laboratory diagnosis of Lyme borreliosis: guidelines from the Canadian Public Health Laboratory Network", Canadian Public Health Network, Can. J. Infect. Dis. Med. Microbiol. 18: 145-148, 2007

symptoms in the disease process. The criterion being used to report Lyme Disease by physicians is often set by state health officials and is often based upon the rigid criteria established by the Center for Disease Control and Prevention (CDC). This CDC criterion was established for an epidemiological survey, which was designed to study the distribution of Lyme Disease.

The wo-step method of the CDC uses a screening immunoassay for all patients followed by a more sensitive and specific Western blot only if the screening test was positive. Unfortunately, this approach was originally intended for *surveillance* of Lyme Disease in potentially asymptomatic patients, not for diagnostic purposes in patients with symptoms that are potentially related to Lyme Disease. This criterion was not intended to be used as a standard for the clinical diagnosis of Lyme Disease; the CDC has clearly stated this. Unfortunately, ignorant health officials and physicians continue to use these criteria for the clinical diagnosis of Lyme Disease.

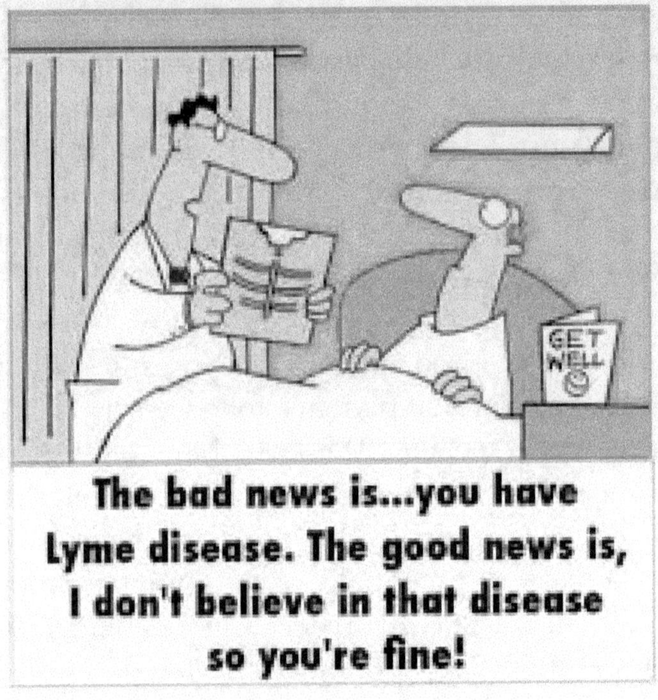


## Problems with Misdiagnosis

The following description of a married couple illustrates the potential seriousness and persistence of increasingly common Lyme and its co-infections and the absolute necessity to receive a proper diagnosis. Virginia T. Sherr, M.D., psychiatrist in private practice in Holland, PA describes these cases. These, as well as case histories similar (possibly yours) demonstrate immediate need for intensive education of all physicians and the public about the risks posed by tick-borne infections. Experiences of these two patients demonstrate necessity for accurate epidemiological reporting of all such vector-borne diseases. Of the titled infections, only Lyme and ehrlichiosis are on the Center of Diseases Control's list of Officially Reportable Diseases.

Descriptions of the patients' symptoms:

## Mr. W's Infection: Unrecognized Chronic Lyme Disease Initiated a Medical Controversy

"Mr. W, an active 76-year-old man (1996) upon his first ever visit to a psychiatrist's office, needed evaluation due to marked changes in his personality. Careful history-taking revealed that he had experienced a rectangular dark red rash on 1 ankle (otherwise asymptomatic) for several weeks circa June 1996. By late that summer, he had gradually developed uncharacteristic and inappropriate outbursts of extreme irritability, altered gait, loss of direction sense, evening chills, episodic daytime sleep urgency, pronounced executive memory loss and variable loss of recent memory. Neurologic and psychiatric workups ensued. In September 1996, his neurologist diagnosed Lyme Disease (LYD) when an enzyme-linked immunosorbent assay blood test revealed a positive IgG of 2.63.

Doxycycline 100 mg twice daily was begun. Mr. W became less symptomatic, his rages abated, and his memory improved. Another specialist, however, questioned accuracy of the diagnosis, terminating the antibiotic after 2 weeks. Axillary lymphadenopathy remained unexplained.

As June 1997 approached, Mr. W's sore left knee was visibly swollen. Nine months after original diagnosis, he also had developed balance problems, strange, shifting, tender, acutely painful areas on his scalp and feet, and a highly distracting, tingling sensation on the tip of his nose. His family physician examined him and confirmed the original diagnosis of persistent, neuro-Lyme Disease.

On 6/3/97, prior to antibiotic treatment, Mr. W suddenly experienced an episode of violent, seizure-like shaking of his entire body, during which he did not lose consciousness.[11] [12] There were no urinary tract or other symptoms. His LYD Western Blot (WB) test (7/9/97) revealed 4 highly significant positive IgG bands plus another: an equivocal band on the same WB test for immune antibodies relating to the causative spirochete, *Borrelia burgdorferi* (Bb).[13]

---

[11] Benach JL, Coleman JL, Habicht GS, et al. Serological evidence for simultaneous occurrences of Lyme Disease and babesiosis. J Infect Dis 1985 Sept;152(3):473-477

[12] Clark IA, Jacobson LS. Do babesiosis and malaria share a common disease process? Ann Trop Med Parasitol 1998 Jun;92(4):483-8

[13] Harris NS. The laboratory's role in the diagnosis of Lyme Disease. In: Folds JD, Nakamura RM, eds. Clinical Diagnostic Immunology: Protocol in Quality Assurance and Standardization. Malden, Mass: Blackwell

Gradually improving but still symptomatic following several months of oral antibiotics, Mr. W's WB immune response increased to show 6 positive, significant, IgG antibody bands against Bb. (4/8/98).

Intensive antibiotic treatment consisted of concomitant oral cefuroxime axetil, cefixime and doxycycline 100 mg three times per day. His knee swelling totally subsided. Later, receiving azithromycin alone, the patient's irritability, disorientation, cognitive problems, and all but 2 other symptoms resolved. He retained his intense need for lengthy daytime naps despite sound nighttime sleep and he experienced episodic afternoon chills despite normal body temperature. He had episodes of dark urine. Diagnostically, however, physicians did not consider babesiosis early on.

When waves of daytime narcoleptic-like sleep attacks and chilliness intensified during evening hours, despite the use of antibiotics, and Mr. W complained that winter's coldness depressed him, he was further evaluated. On 3/26/98, his blood tested positive with a 1:512 indirect fluorescent antibody (IFA) titer for *Babesia microti* at BBI (now "Specialty") Laboratory. His *B microti* polymerase chain reaction (PCR) was also positive (7/7/98) at Medical

Science, 1998:362-382

Diagnostic Laboratories (MDL). Treatment rounds of anti-protozoan medications atovaquone (Mepron) and azithromycin (Zithromax) were undertaken for babesiosis.

## Overview of Mr. W's Follow-Up Laboratory Findings & Treatment of Babesiosis

Fifteen months into treatment by a LYD specialist[14] for chronic babesiosis and LYD, the patient's *B microti* PCR turned negative but his *B burgdorferi* DNA (PCR at MDL) was positive. Mepron was stopped and antibiotic treatment continued. When symptoms resurged in approximately 1 year concomitant with an increasing Human Monocytic Ehrlichiosis (HME) titer, restarting his doxycycline (9/27/00) provided general relief and resolution of lymphadenopathy. However, by April 2001, Mr. W's disorientation, chilliness and sleep urgency intensified once more. His PCR for *B microti* DNA again returned positive, as did his WB for the same organism (MDL).

Because of the positive direct blood test for *B microti* DNA, clinical improvement from LYD symptoms, and the first time fully negative Lyme

---

[14] Bach GP. Antibiotics and atovaquone for Lyme Co-infections: Improvement of Neurologic Signs Including Paralysis. Three Case Reports. Abstract: 12th International Scientific Conference on Lyme Disease and other Spirochetal & Tick-borne Disorders

IgG WB, new emphasis began on re-treatment of chronic babesiosis (5/02). Mr. W received the anti-malarial, Malarone (atovaquone with proquanil), but he also was given a course of dirithromycin (Dynabac) to maintain suppression of likely persistent subclinical borrelial infection. Rationale was that presence of co-infections greatly magnified severity of each. Eventual return of original Lyme disorientation and knee symptoms, however, unveiled resurgences of Lyme WB IgG antibodies (now up to 7 significant bands, 1/30/02—IGeneX Lab) and at MDL, an increase to 3 Babesia antibody bands.[15] At no time did Mr. W need psychotropic medications, other than the stimulant described below.

## Interpretation of Mr. W's Experience with Babesiosis

Mr. W had multiple cycles of treatment with antimicrobial medications (atovaquone, azithromycin, and a combination of atovaquone and proquanil) throughout 4 years with much improvement in memory, affect and general health. Both direct PCR evidence of *Babesia* infection and indirect Babesia tests (increasingly positive antibodies) remained confirmatory of his having active chronic babesiosis. When anti-babesia

---

[15] Krause PJ, Spielman A, Telford SR III, et al. Persistent parasitemia after acute babesiosis. N Engl J Med. 1998;339:160-165

medication lapsed, there were returns to lab and clinical abnormalities.

Persistent daytime sleep urgency despite lengthy antimicrobial treatment, and 6 PM daily chills, may have been residual signs of chronic babesiosis. However, the narcolepsy-like symptom cannot totally be separated from LYD. Direct evidence of both Lyme and babesiosis was still present by positive DNA testing in April 2001 and by increasing antibodies to both in January 2002. Recent intensification of his sleep attacks coincident with current absence of anti-protozoan treatments suggests babesiosis causation. Modafinil (Provigil) 200 mg twice daily greatly improved his wakefulness. Recent developments of positive PCRs for mycoplasma, HHV-6 and a newly developed mild sleep apnea imply possibility of additional causations of his increasing sleep urgency. Of significance, likewise, there are now diminished blood levels of androstenedione, ACTH, ADH and MSH and increased osmolality—a syndrome frequently seen following illness due to chronic neurotoxic diseases[16] such as Lyme Disease and a methicillin-resistant coagulase-negative naso-pharyngeal infection that was diagnosed and treated.

---

[16] Shoemaker RC, Hudnell HK. Possible estuary-associated syndrome: symptoms, vision, and treatment. Environ Health Perspect. 2001;109:539-545

# Mrs. W's Infections, Laboratory Findings & Treatment

Mrs. W's initially unrecognized tick-borne disease manifested neurologically and muscularly. A 66-year-old gardener, she accompanied her husband for evaluation. She described a medically-observed, ring-shaped red rash on the skin of one forearm (1990). At least 3 other similar rashes were observed in the years surrounding that event—2 had the appearance of a *bull's eye*. Seronegative by the ELISA and conventional WB tests, and having no *flu-like symptoms*.

Mrs. W was not considered by specialists to have a treatable tick-borne disease (TBD) until 1997 when chronic neuroborreliosis with multi-system Lyme involvement was diagnosed clinically by her family doctor. Among many symptoms were profound sense of coldness, entire bodily weakness and generalized, painful, severe muscular spasms, cardiac laboring and arrhythmias, waves of painful aural, visual, and touch hypersensitivities, aphonia, a maxillary bone-gum fistula, bradypnea, impatience, multiple sclerosis-like neurological symptoms, chills, and losses of visual acuity. Ocular examination showed a punctate retinal hemorrhage. She appeared on the verge of imminent collapse. Babesiosis originally was not a suspected co-infection.

Mrs. W's intensive 8 months' treatment with intravenous (IV) medications—ceftriaxone followed by IV cefotaxime for treatment of the persistently severe late-stage neuro-LYD symptoms, led to a steady improvement. Attempts to truncate treatment resulted in memory losses and return of muscle pain. She also had received doxycycline 100 mg three times daily for newly resurgent Human Monocytic Ehrlichiosis. Her neurological symptoms, restless legs syndrome, cardiac laboring, unrelenting muscle pains, and generalized weakness slowly lessened but recurred with each attempt to discontinue antibiotics.

Gradual relief continued until January 1998 when treatment for LYD suddenly appeared to falter. While still on IV cefotaxime, symptoms intensified with multiple daily waves of skin flushing, sweating, cardiac arrhythmias, pricking, burning, or searing cutaneous pains, weakness, chills, painful muscle spasms, generalized itching, severe hyperacusis, blurred vision, parched lips, impatience, irritability, clumsiness, insomnia, and exquisite hypersensitivity to touch. Episodic scalp and facial sweating occurred in waves with concomitant late afternoon malaise and episodic chills.

IFA blood tests for *Babesia* then revealed a high titer of 1:512 (BBI). However, Mrs. W was afebrile, with subnormal oral temperatures[17] usually ranging from

---

[17] Wilson ED. Doctor's Manual for Wilson's Syndrome. 3rd ed. Lady

95.7 to 97.0° F Historically, the patient had experienced unexplained blood losses during 2 otherwise uneventful elective surgeries, one preceding and one following this crisis time by several years, although other routine hemograms were consistently normal. Oral iron (300-600 mg/day) restored her postoperative Hgb from 8% to 14.5% each occasion but did not stop profound malaise and episodic chilliness.

## Overview of the Mrs. W's Laboratory Findings and Treatment of Babesiosis

Mrs. W's initial *Babesia* antibody test, negative (1/05/98), was first done many months after IV and oral treatments, including azithromycin, were started to treat her chronic neuroborreliosis (July 1997). She still was being treated for both LYD and ehrlichiosis and symptoms from these were resolving slowly when daily waves of malaise dramatically escalated, incapacitating her in her 8th month of IV antibiotic treatment. Babesiosis was reconsidered diagnostically.

On 3/26/98, IFA tests for *B microti* done at BBI Laboratory revealed the above-mentioned strongly positive babesiosis titer. *Babesia* PCR blood DNA testing also was positive a year later (March 1999, IGeneX Laboratory), following partial treatment

---

Lake, Fla: Muskeegee Medical Publishing, 1997

with atovaquone and azithromycin for her newly recognized chronic babesiosis.[18] [19] Thus, three independent laboratories confirmed positive testing for *B microti*. In addition, a Fluorescent in situ Hybridization (FISH) test (IGeneX) was positive for fluorescing merozoite ring forms of *Babesia* piroplasms. MDL Lab also found Mrs. W's PCR test for Lyme DNA positive (11/8/99). Of additional interest, when the 2 other known diseases were diminished by treatment, there was a return of a variety of symptoms. Ehrlichiosis antibody (HME IgM) titers were then found to have risen to 1:160 (November 1999, IGeneX Lab). Symptomatic relief followed re-treatment with doxycycline. In April 2001, Mrs. W again had evidence of babesiosis via a positive *B microti* WB (MDL). Her Lyme tests now showed 3 significant positive bands on the IgM WB—a known marker for *chronic* as well as acute LYD.[20]

## Interpretation of Mrs. W's Experience

Intensive treatment for babesiosis and Lyme Disease over the span of 4 years returned a handicapped

---

[18] Krause PJ, Lepore T, Sikand VK, et al. Atovaquone and azithromycin for the treatment of babesiosis. N Engl J Med. 2000;343:1454-1458

[19] Allred DR. Babesiosis: Persistence in the face of adversity. TRENDS in Parasitology. 2003Feb;19(2):51-55

[20] Craft JE, Fischer DK, Shimamoto GT, Steere AC. Antigens of Borrelia burgdorferi recognized during Lyme Disease. Appearance of a new immunoglobulin G response late in the illness. J Clin Invest. 1986 Oct;78(4):934-939

Mrs. W to much improved capacity. However, her life still has to be managed around 2-9 milder daily waves of likely *Babesia*-provoked symptoms. Chills subsided *temporarily* when atavoquone and zithromycin were prescribed. Later, as with her husband, a nasopharyngeal culture was positive for the newly discovered neurotoxin-former, methicillin-resistant, coagulase negative *Staphylococcus epidermidis* that had contributed to her discomfort prior to its specific antibiotic treatment.

## Summary of Both Cases

Mr. and Mrs. W, both of whom have documented cases of chronic tick-borne illnesses, including babesiosis, have lived in Pennsylvania most of their lives. Lesions appeared after gardening in their wooded, deer-populated backyard north of Philadelphia. Neither spouse has been re-exposed to ticks.

Both partners have had normal MRIs. However, single-photon emission computed tomography (SPECT) scans of their brains revealed "global heterogeneous hypoperfusion" compatible with impact of noxious influences upon cerebral circulation, cited by the radiologist as likely related to the LYD of each.[21] For one partner

---

[21] Logigian FL, Johnson KA, Kijewski MF. Reversible cerebral hypoperfusion in Lyme encephalopathy. Neurology. 1997;49:1661-1670

microscopically fluorescing intra-erythrocytic parasites were found in 3 widely spaced evaluations.

Neither mate had the acute babesia signs of splenic enlargement or severe hypotension.[22] They were not tested for urinary hemolysis until after atavoquone treatment[23] when these tests were negative. Diagnoses of babesiosis eventually helped to partially explain the inability of both patients to recover fully despite intensive treatment for LYD. Treatment then, for *B microti* infection, sufficiently restored both partners so that they can pursue physical and cognitive activities, although neither is asymptomatic or fully recovered.

## Conclusions

"Lack of general medical awareness of the presence, persistence, and severity of these widely epidemic and backyard-located, spirochetal, rickettsial and protozoan infections caused significant delay in the treatment of this couple. The delay prolonged their illnesses resulting in severe discomfort and long-term disabilities. Early recognition and medical intervention could have prevented much of the ultimate persistence of their infections.[24]

---

[22] Cheng David, Yakobi-Shvlli Rami, Fernandez Jose. Life-threatening hypotension from babesiosis hemolysis. AJEM.
doi:10.1053/ajem.2002.27153
[23] Weiss LM. Babesiosis in humans: a treatment review. Expert Opin Pharmacother. 2002;3:1109-1115
[24] Stricker RB, Lautin A. The Lyme wars: time to listen. Expert Opin

Official recording of *all* vector-borne illnesses in humans needs to be instituted, in order to bring to universal awareness to the true scope of the epidemic and the necessity of proper differentiation and treatment of such infections as Lyme Disease, ehrlichiosis, and babesiosis."[25]

Investig Drugs. 2003;12(10):1609-1614
[25] Two Detailed Case Histories Involving Patients with Co-Infections, by VIRGINIA T. SHERR, M.D., MAY, 2004

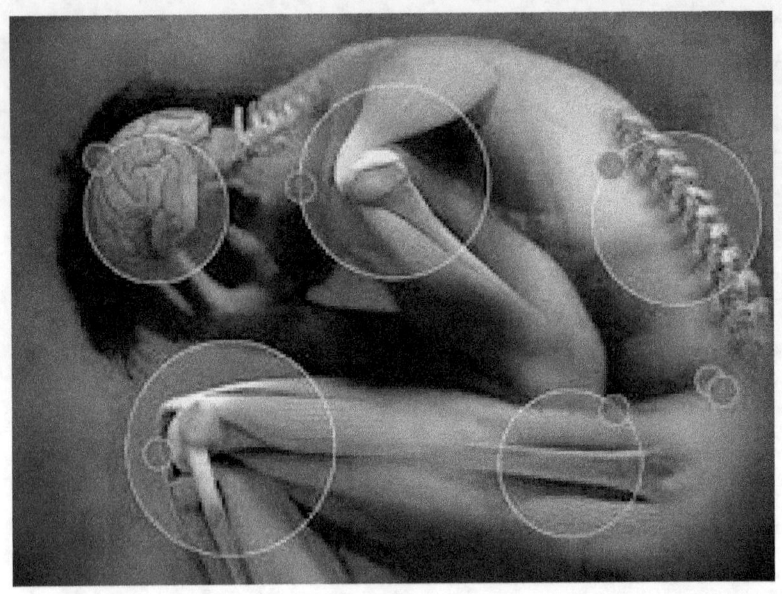

*"Healing is a matter of time, but it is sometimes a matter of opportunity."*
*Hippocrates*

# The Many Faces of Borrelia

Another major oversight by the medical community is that *Borrelia burgdorferi* is the only bacterium that causes Lyme Disease. The truth is that there are many pathogenic Borrelia strains; many of which cause borreliosis (Lyme-like disease); currently I have over 90 Lyme Disease-causing strains in my test kit. The *Borrelia strains* become a type of spirochete when they enter their viral-like phase.

*Borrelia burgdorferi sensu lato* is name given to the overall category. In North America there is just one genospecies variant - *Bb sensu stricto*. In Europe there are three categories Bb sensu stricto, *B. garinii*, and *B. afzelii*. Asia has *B. garinii* and *B. afzelii*. Japan has *B. japonica* and *B. miyamoto*. These groups are evolving as new research discoveries occur.

If it were not difficult enough to get an accurate diagnosis, consider the following:

**There are more carriers of Lyme than just the deer tick.**

There is a tremendous misunderstanding regarding the vector (carrier) that transmits Lyme Disease. First of all, the familiar tick vector called blacklegged ticks (commonly called deer ticks) is more prevalent and widespread than previously reported. Secondly, more evidence supports the belief that ticks are not the only carrier able to transmit Borrelia species including other non-deer ticks and other insects (including mosquitos). Unfortunately, health officials to the public and medical community are not reporting this critical information.

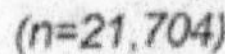

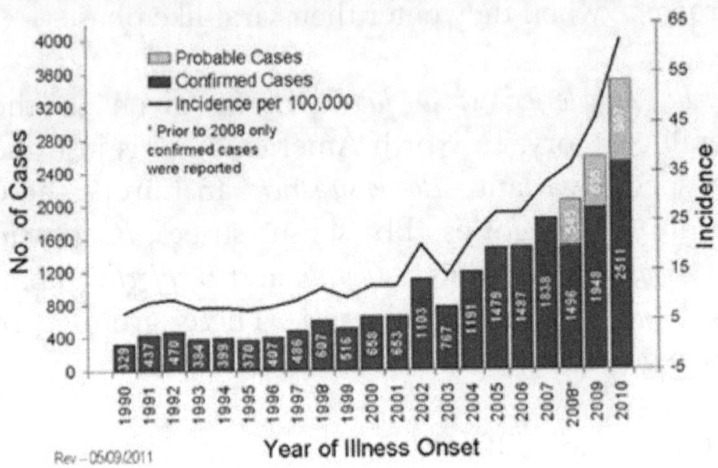



## Lyme is more common than we think.

Health officials are not reporting the true prevalence of Lyme Disease – heck, most "health officials" still argue that it doesn't exist. It is difficult to estimate how many cases are unreported, but it may be 10-15 times higher than what is currently reported. Both self-diagnosed and misdiagnosed cases go unreported (and never become a part of the data) even though Lyme Disease is a mandatory reportable disease in most states.

## Patients need longer and more comprehensive treatment.

The standard therapy of 4 -6 weeks of antibiotic treatment is *only* sufficient to treat Acute, Phase 1

Lyme Disease. Chronic, Phase 2 and 3 Lyme Disease is often a life-long illness that is then just successfully managed (that's what this book is about). These patients end up being diagnosed with psychological disorders, MS, or other autoimmune diseases.

## Wrong diagnosis leads to wrong treatment.

I have **never** been a fan of obtaining a *diagnosis* as most are simply a physician's cop-out to place a name on the set of symptoms. It seems that people are often content with a named diagnosis, even somewhat proud of it. These tend to be the victims in the world, boldly wearing their diagnosis badge and demanding attention for their suffering. May this **never** be you! You cannot allow your struggles to drag you into self-pity and hopelessness. More on this later.

## Lyme Disease is usually accompanied by one or more co-infection.

Take a look at the table below to understand how complex a condition may be. There are multiple possible co-infections that could go along with a diagnosis of Lyme Disease.

| Co-infections | Vector | **Causative Agent** | Endemic Area | Symptoms |
| --- | --- | --- | --- | --- |
| Lyme Disease | Deer Tick<br>Pacific<br>Black-legged Tick | *Borrelia burgdorferi*<br>*Borrelia lonsestari* | Northeast<br>Midwest<br>West Coast | Off season flu<br>Rash (bull's-eye or other)<br>Constitutional symptoms<br>Musculoskeletal symptoms<br>Wide range of neurological symptoms, including Bell's Palsy |
| Babesiosis | Deer Tick<br>Pacific<br>Black-legged Tick | *Babesia microti*<br>*WA-1* | Northeast<br>West Coast | Fever<br>Hemolytic anemia<br>Constitutional symptoms<br>Possible death |
| Ehrlichiosis | Deer Tick<br>Pacific<br>Black-legged tick<br>American Dog Tick<br>Long Star Tick | *Ehrlichia phagocytohphila* | Northeast<br>Upper<br>Midwest | Fever<br>Headache<br>Constitutional symptoms<br>Possible death |
| Colorado Tick Fever | Rocky Mountain Wood Tick | *Colorado Tick Fever Virus* | Western US | Fever with remission<br>Second bout of fever |
| Tick Relapsing Fever | Relapsing fever tick (Ornithodoros turicata) | *Borrelia hermsii* | Western US | Periods of fever<br>Petechial rashes |
| Q Fever | Brown Dog Tick<br>Rocky Mountain Wood Tick<br>Lone Star Tick | *Coxiella burnetii* | Throughout US | Acute fever<br>Chills<br>Sweats |
| Powassan Viral Encephalitis | Woodchuck Tick | *Flavivirus* | Eastern and Western US | Fever<br>Meningoencephalitis<br>10% fatality rate<br>50% Neurological sequela |
| Rocky Mountain Spotted Fever | American Dog Tick<br>Rocky Mountain Wood Tick | *Rickettsia* | Throughout US | Sudden fever<br>Maculopapular rash on soles of hands and feet that spreads over the entire body<br>3%-5% fatality rate |
| Tick Paralysis | American Dog Tick<br>Rocky Mountain Wood Tick<br>Lone Star Tick | *Neurotoxin excreted from tick's salivary gland* | Throughout US | Fatigue<br>Flacid paralysis<br>Tongue and facial paralysis<br>Convulsions<br>Death |
| Tularemia | American Dog Tick<br>Rocky Mountain Wood Tick<br>Lone Star Tick | | Throughout US | Indolent ulcers<br>Swollen lymph nodes<br>Deaths can occur |
| Bartonella | Cats<br>Ticks<br>Fleas | *Bartonella Quintana*<br>*Bartonella henselea* | Worldwide | Fever<br>Mild neurological signs<br>Granulomatous lymphadenitis<br>Red popular lesion |

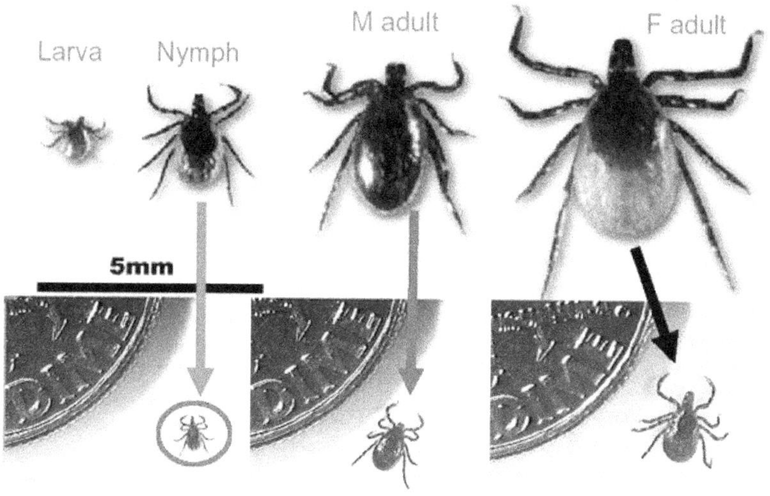


## The question on everyone's mind: "How do I know which Phase I am in?"

In my desire to help everyone regardless of his or her ability to pay for care, I've assembled a few criteria on our website to help you determine your phase at
**ConnersClinic.com/your-lyme-phase**

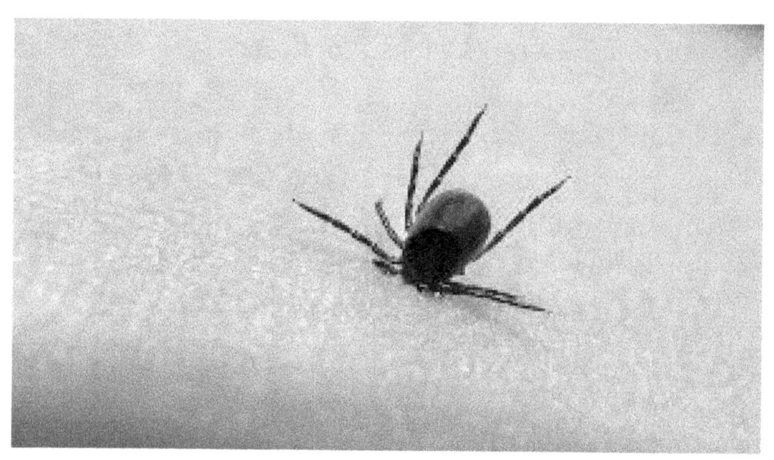

# THE HISTORY AND PROGRESSIVE UNDERSTANDING OF LYME DISEASE

According to Adams Medical Encyclopedia, "Lyme Disease was first reported in the United States in the town of Old Lyme, Connecticut, in 1975." In the United States, most Lyme Disease infections occur in the following areas:

- Northeastern states, from Virginia to Maine
- North-Central states, mostly in Wisconsin and Minnesota
- West Coast, particularly northern California

Risk factors for Lyme Disease include:

- Doing outside activities that increase tick exposure (for example, gardening, hunting, or hiking) in an area where Lyme Disease is known to occur
- Having a pet that may carry ticks home
- Walking in high grasses

Important facts about tick bites and Lyme Disease:

- In most cases, a tick must be attached to your body for 24 - 36 hours to spread the bacteria to your blood.
- Blacklegged ticks can be so small that they are almost impossible to see. Many people with Lyme Disease never even saw a tick on their body.
- Most people who are bitten by a tick do not get Lyme Disease.

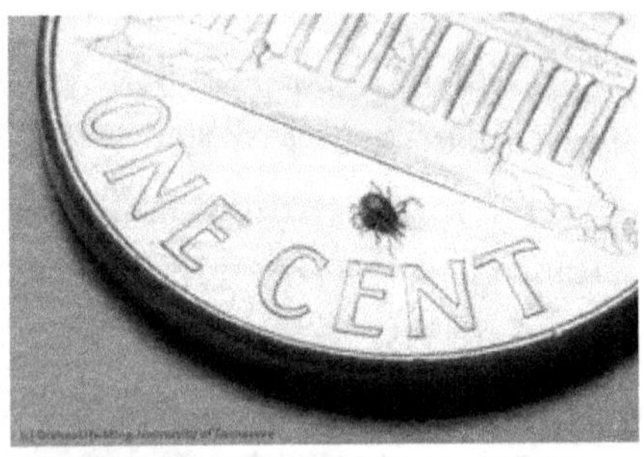

See videos on our website for further clarification at **ConnersClinic.com/lyme**

# How Lyme Hides - First, Our Own Microbes

Beginning immediately at birth, humans are colonized by a myriad of microorganisms that assemble into complex stereotypic communities, creating a beneficial indigenous microbiota (our flora). The result is a *supra-organism* in which our microbial partners outnumber our human cells by 10-to-1. Most currently available information about the human microbiota concerns the bacterial component, although they are by no means the only important members. However, bacteria will be the focus of this discussion.

In contrast to the relatively rare harmful encounters with pathogens (like Lyme), indigenous human-microbe relationships are the dominant forms in which we interact with microbes and are fundamentally important to human physiology. Co-adaptation and co-dependency are features of our relationships with these friendly bugs.

## This we now know to be true:

- The human microbiota facilitates nutrient acquisition and energy extraction from food,
- It promotes terminal (postnatal) differentiation of mucosal structure and function, and
- It stimulates both the innate and adaptive immune

systems.

By so, being the primary stimulation of immune system function, it helps to create an epithelial boundary and integrity, as well as to *educate* our innate immune defenses. It also provides *colonization resistance* against pathogen invasion, regulates intermediary metabolism, and processes ingested chemicals.

It also is extremely important in the resistance of Lyme Disease. Symbiotic microbiota resist all pathogenic species simply by competing with territory. Unfortunately, Lyme bacteria migrate to places our normal microbes dare not go. Intracellular (within the cell) penetration is one such place but, by all means, it is not the only way Lyme evades immune destruction.

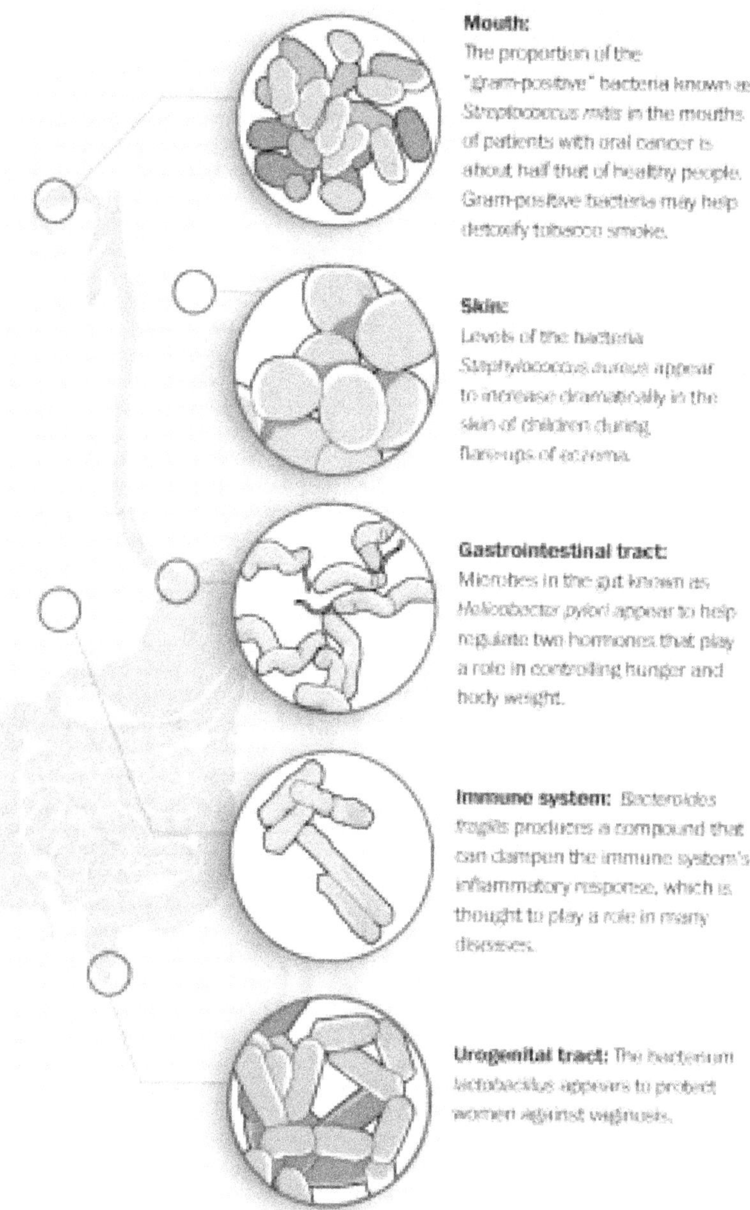


Precisely how our microbial community is assembled is still just being better studied. In the neonatal period, the community assembly process is especially dynamic and is influenced by early environmental (in particular, maternal) exposures. It is believed that the composition and functional capabilities of the indigenous microbiota evolve in a generally orderly fashion, as diet, hormonal environment, other environmental factors, and occasional ecologic disturbances play out their effects on a distinct, albeit diverse, human genetic background.

Differences in the capability of strains may explain variation among individuals in the metabolism of drugs such as digoxin and other exogenous chemicals as well as an individual's ability to fight off virulent pathogens. Differences in the capability of strains to tolerate normal inflammation may also influence the composition of the microbiota. Although there is evidence for shared functional capabilities among the intestinal microbial communities of different healthy humans, host genetics is a source of variation in the makeup of the human indigenous microbiota.

## What is an Infection?

*Infection* (or *colonization*) is simply the establishment of a microorganism on or within a host; it may be short lived, as in our encounters with *transients*, or be persistent and may result in only low gain or harm to either participant.

*H.pylori* would be another example. While it *may* cause immediate disease (stomach ulcers), it may also lead to chronic, insidious, subclinical effects with long-term consequences (cancer, heart disease). Many microorganisms with a capacity for sustained multiplication in humans, including members of the indigenous microbiota, cause disease more readily in individuals with underlying chronic disease or in those who are otherwise compromised. The common term *opportunist* suits this category of pathogen well.

What are the distinguishing characteristics of microbes that live in humans? A successful Lyme pathogen must do the following:

- Enter the human host,
- Become established, which includes successful competition with indigenous microbes,
- Acquire nutrients,
- Avoid or circumvent the host's innate defenses and a powerful immune system,
- Above all, replicate,
- Disseminate, if necessary, to a preferred site, and

Eventually, **all** pathogens desire to be transmitted to a new susceptible host.

## The Genes

Whether a pathogen or a commensal, a microorganism must also possess an interactive group of complementary genetic properties that promote its interaction with the human host. For a given microorganism, the genetic traits define unique attributes that enable it to follow a common sequence of steps used in establishing infection or, in some cases, subsequent disease.

Genetic testing techniques now permit the identification, isolation, and characterization of many of these genes. The availability of the host (e.g. human) genome sequence also enables multiple synergistic approaches for understanding virulence, including the identification of host susceptibility traits, genome-wide assessments of host response, and clues about the mechanisms of host defense and pathogen counter-defense.

## Smart Bugs

It has long been but a hypothesis that pathogens (take *Borellia* from Lyme for example) breach intact host anatomic, cellular, or biochemical barriers that ordinarily prevent entry by other microorganisms. Thus, pathogens "go where other microbes dare not." In addition, many pathogens, such as *Borellia*, *Mycobacterium tuberculosis*, *Treponema pallidum*, *Chlamydia trachomatis*, and *Salmonella typhi*, have the

50

capacity to establish persistent (often subclinical) infection in the human host and have evolved the extraordinary capacity to live in the inner sanctums of our innate and adaptive immune defenses or, in general, to compete well in the face of otherwise hostile host conditions.

Some may even evoke human macrophage activity to defend itself against immune attack!

For example, *Salmonella* profits from the inflammatory response that it provokes in the gut by using the oxidized form of a locally produced host factor for a selective growth advantage against commensals. A distinction, then, between a primary pathogen and opportunist is that the pathogen has an *inherent* ability to breach the host barriers that ordinarily restrict other microbes, whereas the opportunist requires some underlying defect or alteration in the host's defenses, whether it be genetic, ecologic (altered microbiota), or caused by underlying disease, to establish itself in a usually privileged host niche. Clearly, the nature of the host plays as important a role as the pathogen in determining outcome.

An initial step required of a pathogen is to gain access to the host in sufficient numbers. Such access requires that the microorganism not only make contact with an appropriate surface but also then reach its *unique* niche or microenvironment on or within the host. This requirement is not trivial.

51

Some pathogens must survive for varying periods in the external environment. Others have evolved an effective and efficient means of transmission. To accomplish this goal, the infecting microbe may make use of motility, chemotactic properties, and adhesive structures (or *adhesins*) that mediate binding to specific eukaryotic cell receptors or to other microorganisms (piggybacking on other microbes).

Pathogens that persist at the surface of skin or mucosa usually rely upon multiple redundant adhesins and adherence mechanisms. If the adhesin is immunogenic, expression is usually regulated; in addition, antigenic variants may arise. Preexisting microorganisms (the host's existing microbiota) provide competition against establishment of the newcomer so long as it is healthy and abundant.

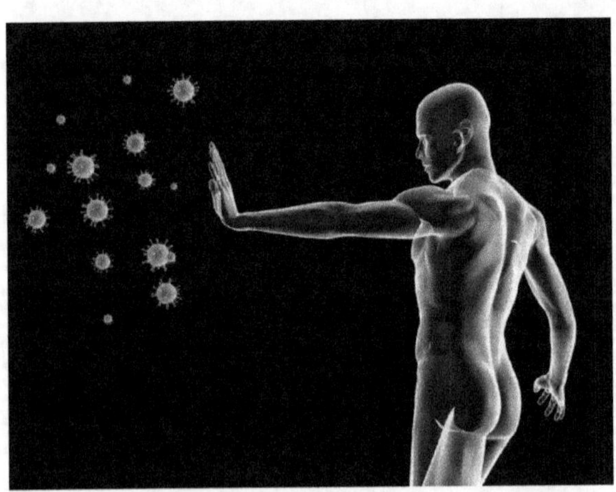

Normal inherent host defense mechanisms should pose the most difficult set of obstacles for pathogens and commensals in establishing themselves in a host.

For any set of specific host defenses, an individual pathogen will have a unique and distinctive counterstrategy. Some of the best-known mechanisms that pathogenic microbes use for countering host defenses include the use of an antiphagocytic capsule and the elaboration of toxins and microbial enzymes that act on host immune cells and/or destroy anatomic barriers. These are smart bugs, after all.

Microorganisms also use subtle biochemical mechanisms to avoid, subvert, or, as we now increasingly understand, manipulate host defenses. These strategies include the elaboration of immunoglobulin-specific proteases, iron sequestration mechanisms, coating themselves with host proteins to confuse the immune surveillance system, or causing host cells to signal inappropriately, leading to dysregulation of host defenses or even host cell death. It really is quite amazing!

Examples of these mechanisms include the production of immunoglobulin A1 protease by the meningococci, the use of receptors for iron-saturated human transferrin and lactoferrin by *N. gonorrhoeae*, and the coating of *T. pallidum* with human soluble fibronectin.

*Yersinia*, *Mycobacterium*, and *Bordetella* stimulate a TH2 response and diminish the killer cells by inducing host cell production of interleukin-10, which is a

53

potent immunosuppressive cytokine so it can slip past defense like a cunning spy. Antigenic variation and intracellular invasion are other common strategies used by successful pathogens to avoid immune detection.

## Their Ultimate Purpose

The ability to multiply is a characteristic of all living organisms since, ultimately, reproduction and survival is its goal. Whether the pathogen's habitat in the relevant host is intracellular or extracellular, mucosal or submucosal, within the bloodstream or within another privileged anatomic site, pathogens have evolved a distinct set of biochemical tactics to achieve this goal. The ultimate success of a pathogen, indeed, of any microorganism, is measured by the degree to which it can multiply and to the extent that it succeeds is to the demise of the host.

An emerging concept of microbial disease causation, with origins in the field of ecology, is the notion of "community as pathogen," in which a conserved broad feature of the microbial community contributes to pathology, rather than any one specific member or component. This concept may be relevant to a wide variety of chronic inflammatory processes of skin and mucosa, including inflammatory bowel disease and chronic periodontitis. This concept answers questions many clinicians may have encountered as to the difficultly in both isolating and treating an individual pathogen.

In addition, microbial pathogenesis involves synergies between organisms, as well as between gene products, each of which may be insufficient alone in causing disease. For example, several members of the human health-associated nasopharyngeal microbiota, including *Streptococcus pneumoniae*, *Neisseria meningitidis*, and *Streptococcus pyogenes*, regularly cause well-defined, well-known human diseases. You may develop antibodies to individual organisms, yet such commensal pathogens persist in a significant proportion and can be associated with both acute and chronic disease.

# Summary

## How Lyme avoids being killed by your immune system (phagocytosis)

1. Lyme **hides**. The pathogens may invade or remain confined in regions inaccessible to phagocytes inside of cells and/or in certain internal tissues (e.g. the lumens of glands, the urinary bladder) and surface tissues (e.g.

unbroken skin) that are not well patrolled by phagocytes.

2. Lyme bacteria may be able to ***avoid provoking an overwhelming inflammatory response***. Without inflammation the host is unable to focus the phagocytic defenses.

3. Lyme bacteria or their products ***inhibit phagocyte chemotaxis***. For example, they suppress neutrophil chemotaxis, that is, they prevent an immune cells ability to be chemically attracted to it. This is an extremely handy spy technique that basically fools your immune system into thinking that the Lyme bacteria are the *good guys*.

4. Lyme ***disguises*** itself. Lyme pathogens can cover their surface with a component which is seen as *self* by the host immune system. Such a strategy hides the antigenic surface of the bacterial cell. Phagocytes cannot recognize it upon contact and the possibility of the B cells creating antibodies to enhance phagocytosis is minimized.

5. Lyme bacteria may employ strategies to ***avoid engulfment*** (ingestion) if immune cells do make contact with them. This is not an uncommon strategy as many important pathogenic bacteria bare on their surfaces substances that inhibit phagocytic adsorption or engulfment. Classic examples of antiphagocytic substances on bacterial surfaces include polysaccharide capsules and biofilms with different proteins.

6. Lyme bacteria may possess the cunning ability to **_meld their DNA_** with symbiotic microbiota to completely morph its frequency and appear as a part of the host's microbiota.

**_Bottom line – Lyme stays alive through ingenious methods to replicate and make your life miserable._**

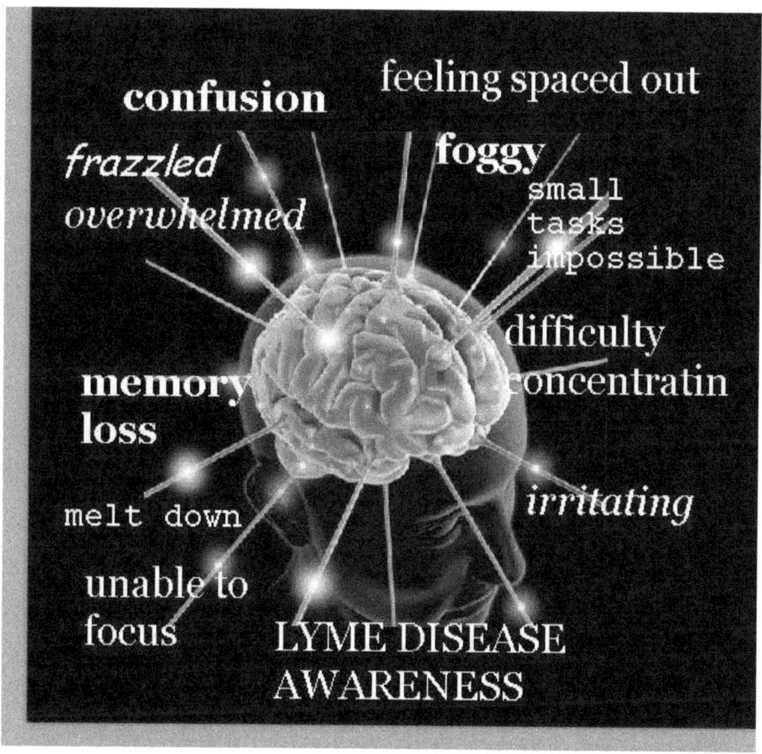

# How Lyme Attacks the Brain & Understanding the Blood-Brain Barrier

Because some of the most damaging and debilitating symptoms of Lyme affect the nervous system, particularly the brain, it is important to understand how this happens. Note: see my book *Lyme Brain* for more detail on this subject.

The blood-brain-barrier (BBB) is a feature of our anatomy and physiology. There are specialized cells in our bodies that act as a blocking wall or filter, which prevents many substances from getting into our brains and spinal cord. The BBB makes it impossible, or at least very tough, for medications to reach the brain (which is mostly a good thing—we don't want chemicals in our brains!)

Throughout our bodies, we have capillaries (our smallest blood vessels), which have a lining of specialized cells (endothelial). These endothelial cells are tightly fitted together to form a filter, which protects the brain by preventing large molecules from passing through to it. Your BBB can be weakened by various illnesses, radiation, infection, and trauma.[26]

---

[26] THE CELL BIOLOGY OF THE BLOOD-BRAIN BARRIER, Annual Review of Neuroscience, Vol. 22: 11-28 (Volume publication date March 1999)DOI: 10.1146/annurev.neuro.22.1.11 L. L. Rubin Ontogeny, Inc., Cambridge, Massachusetts 02138-1118

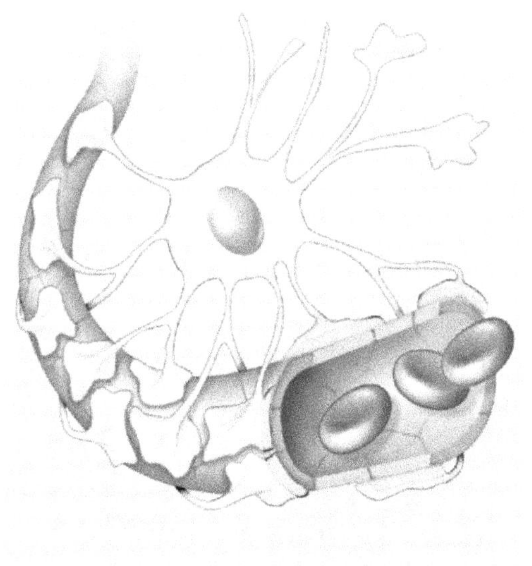

The BBB, which is formed by the endothelial cells that line cerebral micro vessels and specialized glial (brain) cells called astrocytes, have an important role in maintaining a precisely regulated microenvironment for reliable neuronal signaling in the brain. This means that when an organism like Lyme infiltrates the brain by passing through a damaged BBB, all sorts of bad things can happen. Most assuredly, the patient will have a local (in the brain) inflammatory process that, depending on the precise location, will alter normal neuronal conduction and mimic gross lesions. Long-term inflammation is a cause of gross lesions that then are commonly diagnosed as the disorder displayed.[27]

---

[27] Nature Reviews Neuroscience 7, 41-53 (January 2006) | doi:10.1038/nrn1824

59

For example, at present there are approximately 2.1 million people that have a diagnosis of Multiple Sclerosis in America. Symptoms of MS are unpredictable; vary from person to person, and from time to time in the same person. For example: One person may experience abnormal fatigue and episodes of numbness and tingling. Another could have loss of balance and muscle coordination making walking difficult. Still another could have slurred speech, tremors, stiffness, and bladder problems.

Sometimes major symptoms disappear completely, and the person regains lost functions. In severe MS, people have symptoms on a permanent basis including partial or complete paralysis, and difficulties with vision, cognition, speech, and elimination.[28]

Just like many of our *disease diagnoses*, a diagnosis of MS tells you nothing of the cause! Can Lyme be the cause of MS? Of course, it can! Is Lyme always the cause of MS? Of course not!

Furthermore, brain inflammation from Lyme is not dependent on the Lyme spirochete itself crossing the BBB. Inflammation elsewhere in the body is defined by the release of specialized chemicals called cytokines. There are specific cytokines that are

---

[28] http://www.nationalmssociety.org/about-multiple-sclerosis/what-we-know-about-ms/faqs-about-ms/index.aspx#howmany

highly inflammatory and are proven to cross the
BBB.[29]

Antibiotic drugs are typically too large to cross the
BBB. And, if they do get through, it is thought that
they cannot penetrate in large enough quantity to
have the desired effect. This makes infections of the
brain difficult to treat. Although weakening of the
BBB may make it possible for some antibiotics to
break through, it is highly questionable whether or
not it is safe for them to get there!

If the patient is **not** Phase 3 (Autoimmune), herbal
remedies such as teasel, cat's claw, or samento, may
be good for Lyme. While some people have found
them symptomatically helpful, their molecules
cannot cross the BBB either and can leave the
patient frustrated from their ongoing neurological
symptoms.

***Note: The blood-brain-barrier is not a factor
when it comes to homeopathic whole-body,
Rife frequency healing, and some other
wellness-based approaches to healing.***

Comprehensive          homeopathy          and          Rife
are *energy medicine*, not chemical approaches. Many
highly reputable medical sources concur that energy
medicine is a big part of the future of health care.

---

[29] Passage of Cytokines across the Blood-Brain Barrier, Banks W.A..a ·
Kastin A.J.a · Broadwell R.D.b

The truth is that it has already been widely available, but not accepted or pursued by the masses in traditional Western medicine.

If you have been on antibiotics for years in an effort to recover from Lyme, perhaps you will want to consider this information wisely. If Lyme Borrelia bacteria, as well as Bartonella, Ehrlicia, and Babesia are living in your brain, can antibiotics likely kill them? This question does not even take into account the antibiotic resistant nature of many bacteria species.

# H. pylori, a Common Co-Infection

Your gut is a barrier. When we eat food, the pathogens that may accompany the food hit the first barrier; the stomach acid present to digest also prevents infection. Here, the pH is extremely acidic for two main reasons: it breaks down food to be absorbed and kills pathogens trying to hitch a ride. This second purpose of HCl (stomach acid) is of vital importance as it is the first line of defense against potential destroyers of other barriers like the BBB.

Helicobacter pylori (H. pylori), for example, are ubiquitous bacteria that should be easily killed by a normal acid balance in the stomach. If you have an imbalanced HCl supply, H. pylori infiltrates and can either cause a stomach or duodenal ulcer or will pass through attacking other organs. It is estimated that 95% of H. pylori infections are chronic, insidious and subclinical – meaning it is rarely diagnosed as a disorder itself and usually the culprit of many other named diseases. H. pylori is such a common cause of vessel damage that leads to both heart disease and **BBB** disruption that we *must* address it in a book about Lyme since one hypothesis states that one way Lyme survives is to bind itself (through the DNA) to H. pylori.

If Lyme co-hides with H. Pylori, how does it enter the brain? It does so through the blood vessels. More specifically, through the cells that line the vessels called endothelial cells.

Under normal conditions, chemicals released by tissues knock on the endothelial cell's door looking for permission to enter. For instance, a sympathetic nervous system response (fight or flight) in the brain to a perceived stress causes the release of a chemical that will enter a gate in the endothelial fence to cause the smooth muscle layer to contract and narrow the lumen of the vessel. This increases the speed of blood flow and increases the blood pressure so you can run away from the danger. It is a normal response, but like any normal response, we can get *stuck* in an *on* position from chronic source of stimulation.

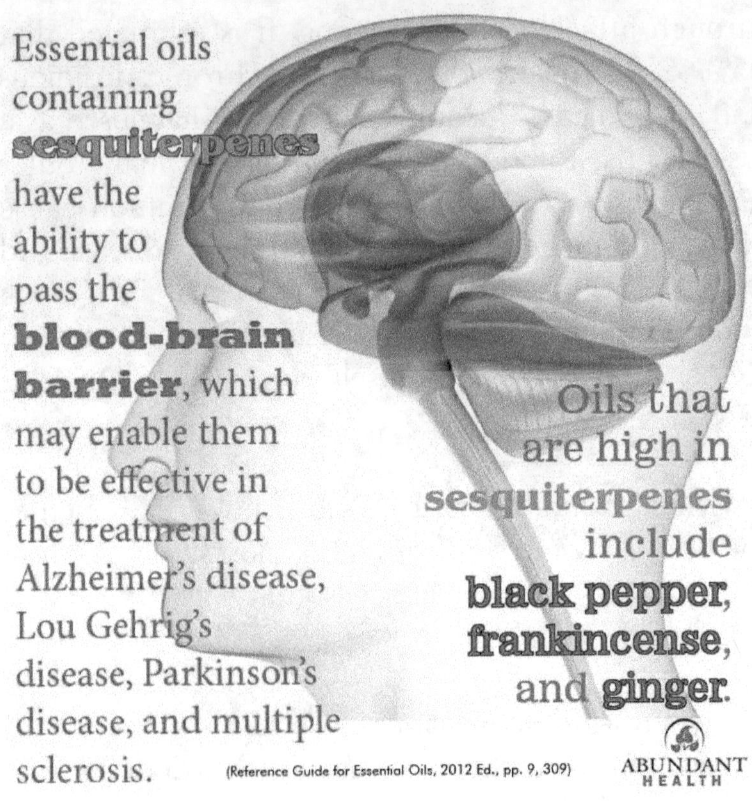


There are really an endless number of possible insults that could *breach the gates* of the endothelial wall – Lyme is just **one** of these. Chemical toxicity, heavy metal toxicity, food additives, flavorings, colorings, infections, and endotoxins are just a few of the other things that can break the gates and cause damage to the endothelial layer (the small, smooth muscles and tissue underneath) and interact with the astrocytes that act as the next (and special) barrier in the brain. You may have heard about the damage that Homocysteine, glucose, or oxidized LDL cause, but by far, the worst culprit for damage is infection. Subclinical (silent) infections (like H. pylori and Lyme) are the number one *bad guy* causing endothelial disease, which leads to BBB disruption (among other things). "Subclinical" means the patient doesn't know they have it! It's a silent disorder that can cause mild, insidious vasculature damage for years (and yes, it can start at birth) until the victim has symptoms of ADHD, anxiety, depression, memory loss and dementia, just to name a few. I know this is a lot of info, so I'll sum this up:

1. BBB disruption really starts with damage to the endothelial layer – the single-celled barrier that lines the vessels.
2. If the endothelial layer is breached, several bad things occur that lead to inflammation in the vessel wall, the tiny muscles underneath the wall, and the astrocyte cells that are meant to keep larger molecules of things out of the CNS.
3. Many possible sources of endothelial damage exist due to poor diet, environmental exposure to toxins, and ubiquitous infectious organisms but subclinical infections (unknown to the patient) are the most common and least diagnosed cause of endothelial disease and hence, brain disorders.

Endothelial disease is always the start of BBB disruption and usually never addressed by any doctor. Heck, most doctors don't even address the fact that there is a disruption in the **BBB**. Worse, many doctors are still blaming the patient's depression on a chemical imbalance as if it were a disease that the poor victim contracted when they were caught out in the rain without a jacket. Medications can change a person's mood, they can numb symptoms, and dull hyperactivity. Medications cannot cure because they do nothing for cause.

## The Three Responses in the Endothelial Cells

There are three possible responses that occur when vascular endothelium is damaged by the infinite number of possible insults:

- a local inflammatory response,
- an oxidative stress response,
- and an autoimmune reaction.

All three may eventually occur and all include inflammation, which is the more damaging aspect of each response. Like every tissue, the endothelium maintains a fine balance between injury and repair. It's like a teeter-totter that tips gently back and forth; vessels are damaged by endless assaults and then healed by a collection of innate physiologic responses that viewed as a whole, over time, we call health. If an individual has the unfortunate event of continual and prolonged damage, the repair can actually bring about problems that we shall soon see.

For fear that I've already bored you to tears, I'll just summarize my point here:

**Over time, a ramped-up immune response involved in Chronic Lyme does a multitude of things:**

1. It destroys endothelial tissue (both receptors and entire cells) due to collateral damage in its attempts to kill the antigen, and
2. It starts to mistake self-tissue for the enemy and begins direct destruction of self-tissue, and
3. An immune response can destroy the astrocyte barrier further allowing antigens to enter the CNS and further the inflammatory spread *inside the brain*!

# Review of the 3 Phases of Lyme

## Phase 1: Acute Infection

In this phase, the patient *still has the capability to kill the disease with an antibiotic*. This is why I highly recommend that those living in Lyme-infested areas have antibiotics on hand to use, should they develop

67

symptoms in Lyme season. *This is only open for a window of time!*

*The* window of opportunity *to* kill *Lyme in the Acute Phase can be very short.*

## Phase 2: Chronic Lyme

Chronic Lyme phase begins the moment the first bacteria *exit* the bloodstream and *enter* the intracellular space (go inside the cell and hide.) This phase still may be treated with antibiotics and immune-boosting nutraceuticals, but it will be a *long, drawn-out treatment plan.* Though it is better than Phase 3, Chronic Lyme is horrible.

## Phase 3: Autoimmune Lyme

When the patient's condition continues to linger, the immune system is constantly trying to kill it. In doing so, the *killer* side of the immune system, the Th1 response, fires to kill the pathogen. When it cannot find the hiding Lyme, the B-cell (Th2) response fires to create antibodies to *tag* the bacteria in order to make them easier to recognize by the killer (Th1) cells. After months of teetering back and forth from a Th1-Th2 reaction, the B cells begin to create antibodies against *your own cells*. This is the very definition of an autoimmune disease and is exactly what takes place in Phase 3 Lyme.

*Now that you have antibodies to self-tissue, every time you fire an immune response for* **any** *reason, or take immune stimulants to* **boost your immune system**, *you are* **killing yourself first***!*

These patients are miserable, and it is the Autoimmune Phase of Lyme that is deadly.

# Neurological Symptoms of Phase 2 & 3

Phase 2 & 3 Lyme patients, due to inflammation in the brain from either systemic inflammation or direct infiltration of spirochetes across the blood-brain barrier, may experience a number of neurological symptoms.

Initially, most people think of swollen and painful joints when they think of Lyme Disease, if they think of anything at all. However, when you look at the symptom list below, you can see that every part of the body can be affected. The frightening collection of neurological symptoms experienced by many Lyme Disease patients is frequently called "neuro-Lyme", but in fact only represents a portion of the illness.

# Do you have any of these symptoms?

**Head, Face, Neck:**
- Unexplained hair loss
- Headache (mild or severe)
- Twitching of facial or other muscles
- Facial paralysis (Bell's palsy)
- Tingling of nose, cheek, or face
- Stiff or painful neck, creaks and cracks
- Jaw pain or stiffness
- Sore throat

**Eyes/Vision:**
- Double or blurry vision
- Increased floating spots
- Pain in eyes, or swelling around eyes
- Oversensitivity to light
- Flashing lights
- Ears/Hearing
- Decreased hearing in one or both ears
- Buzzing in ears
- Pain in ears, oversensitivity to sound
- Ringing in one or both ears

**Digestive and Excretory Systems:**
- Diarrhea
- Constipation
- Irritable bladder (trouble starting, stopping)
- Upset stomach (nausea or pain)

**Musculoskeletal System:**

- Any joint pain or swelling
- Stiffness of joints, back, neck
- Muscle pain or cramps

**Respiratory and Circulatory Systems:**
- Shortness of breath, cough
- Chest pain or rib soreness
- Night sweats or unexplained chills
- Heart palpitations or extra beats
- Heart blockage

**Neurological System:**
- Tremors or unexplained shaking
- Burning or stabbing sensations in the body
- Weakness or partial paralysis
- Pressure in the head
- Numbness in body, tingling, pinpricks
- Poor balance, dizziness, difficulty walking
- Increased motion sickness
- Lightheadedness, wooziness

**Psychological Well-being:**
- Mood swings, irritability
- Unusual depression
- Disorientation (getting or feeling lost)
- Feeling as if you are losing your mind
- Over-emotional reactions, crying easily
- Too much sleep or insomnia
- Difficulty falling or staying asleep

**Mental Capacity:**
- Memory loss (short or long term)
- Confusion, difficulty in thinking

- Difficulty with concentration or reading
- Going to the wrong place
- Speech difficulty (slurred or slow)
- Stammering speech
- Forgetting how to perform simple tasks

**Reproduction and Sexuality:**
- Loss of sex drive
- Sexual dysfunction

**Females Only:**
- Unexplained menstrual pain, irregularity
- Unexplained breast pain, discharge
- Pelvic pain

**General Well-Being:**
- Unexplained weight gain or loss
- Extreme fatigue
- Swollen glands
- Unexplained fevers (high- or low-grade)
- Continual infections (sinus, kidney, eye, etc.)
- Symptoms seem to change, come and go
- Pain migrates (moves) to different body parts
- Early on, experienced a flu-like illness, after which you have not since felt well

So, how do we test for this and how do we treat it? We'll explain these in the next sections.

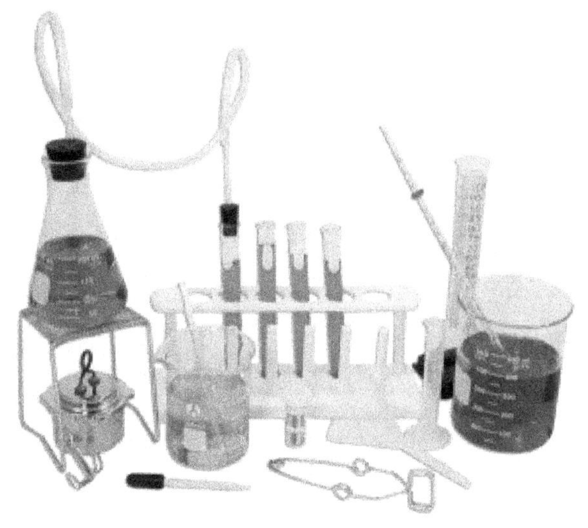

# CONNERS CLINIC CLEAR LYME PROTOCOLS & TREATMENT OPTIONS

We understand that many of you have suffered in silence and have exhausted your finances. This is why we provide this book as a free download on our website with links to many videos, and we give away all of our treatment protocols for free. Our clinic does accept Lyme patients occasionally, but we are so busy with cancer patients that we have a limit to what we can do. So, the more I can empower you, the better.

# How do you test for Lyme if you just don't know if you have it?

## Standard Lab Testing

What does the CDC say? According to the Center of Disease Control (CDC), they recommend a two-step testing procedure when testing blood for evidence of antibodies against the Lyme Disease bacteria. Both steps can be done using the same blood sample:

"The first step uses a testing procedure called 'EIA' (enzyme immunoassay) or rarely, an 'IFA' (indirect immunofluorescence assay). If this first step is negative, no further testing of the specimen is recommended. If the first step is positive or indeterminate (sometimes called 'equivocal'), the second step should be performed. The second step uses a test called an immunoblot test, commonly, a 'Western blot' test. Results are considered positive only if the EIA/IFA and the immunoblot are both positive.

The two steps of Lyme Disease testing are designed to be done together. CDC does not recommend skipping the first test and just doing the Western blot. Doing so will increase the frequency of false positive results and may lead to misdiagnosis and improper treatment.

New tests may be developed as alternatives to one or both steps of the two-step process. Before CDC will recommend new tests, their performance must be demonstrated to be equal to or better than the results of the existing procedure, and they must be FDA approved." (From the CDC website)

**Let's cut to the chase because I totally disagree with the CDC and think it's ridiculous.**

Why? Because if you have symptoms that lead you to believe that you *possibly* have Acute Lyme, by the time the tests come back, you may already have missed the window of treatment!

**Enough of the CDC nonsense, here's real life:**

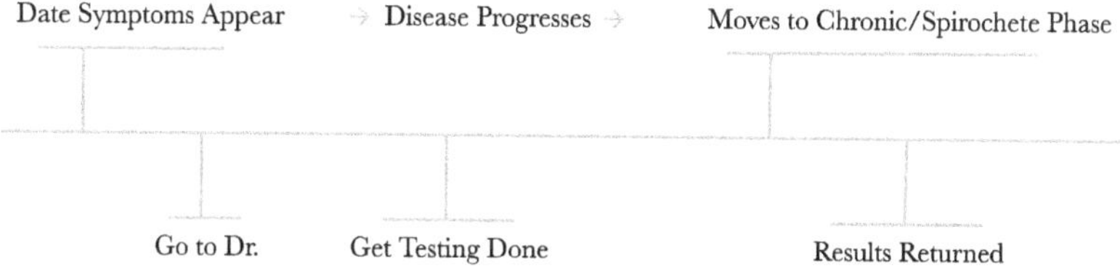


Even *if* the tests performed were optimally accurate, the results usually are returned *after* the window of opportunity to treat the disease with something as simple as antibiotics passes!

This *window of opportunity* is different in length with everyone! I've seen Acute Lyme progress to Phase 2 Lyme in a matter of days; others may be lucky enough to have weeks. This fact forces me to respectfully decline the CDC's above protocol and I think it would be prudent for you to follow suit.

## Other Lab Tests

If you know that you are already beyond Phase 1 and just want to confirm that you have Lyme:

### IgenX Lab (see IgenX.com)

IgenX Lab offers the following tests according to their information:
- The Lyme IFA Test (a piece of the Lyme Panel) – detects IgG, IgM, and IgA antibodies against B. burgdorferi.
- IgM Testing – These tend to be present after about a month following initial infection and are often elevated throughout the disease.
- Western Blot – This is a piece of the CDC recommendation and is possibly the most commonly ordered Lyme test. It is often a false negative and this has caused numerous patients relying on this test alone to be erroneously given improper care leaving them to suffer the consequences.

- The Lyme Dot Assay (LDA) – This looks for pieces of bacteria in the urine. They claim that the specificity is greater than 90% but I doubt this.
- The Polymerase Chain Reaction test (PCR) – This is a highly specific and fairly sensitive test to detect the DNA of the Lyme bacteria. This is often the only marker that may be found on the patient. The problem is that it does ***not*** measure the presence of co-infections. It can be done with a sample of serum, urine or CSF.

## Lyme and Co-Infection DNA Test

We currently use a DNA Lyme Panel test that tests for many different genes that are found in Borrelia burgdorferi, the most common cause of Lyme Disease in the United States, and many common Lyme Disease co-infectors including *Babesia microti, Babesia divergens, Babesia duncani, Bartonella bacilliformis, Bartonella henselae, Bartonella quintanta, Borrelia miyamotoi, Borrelia recurrentis, Ehrlichia chaffensis and Anaplasma phagocytophilum.* Testing of Lyme co-infectors (other tick-transmitted organisms) indicates likely infection with the Lyme spirochete as well.

A positive PCR result from the DNA Connexions Lyme test indicates the presence of DNA from B. burgdorferi and/or other co-infectors. A negative result does not prove a patient is not infected with a tick-borne infection, rather it indicates the absence of detectable Lyme and/or other tick-borne co-infections. A patient's ability to fight the disease, stage of infection, and timing of courses of antibiotics are only some of the factors that may affect the detectability of the spirochete's DNA.

See a sample report at
**ConnersClinic.com/dna-lyme-test**

## If I Do Get Tested, Which Test is the Best?

Here's my take:

1. If you ***need*** lab proof (for whatever reason) – Use the DNA Connexions Test available from any clinician who signs up with the lab (or try to contact the lab themselves at dnsconnexions.com) OR the IGenX Lab (contact the lab directly for this test) to ***prove*** Lyme. Use Cyrex Lab (Array 10) available through our office to ***prove*** autoimmune antibodies.

2. Many people can forgo a test if they have enough signs and symptoms to conclude Lyme and/or its many co-infections may be involved. A clinical conclusion is often

necessary and justified to save both time and money.

## Clinical Evaluation

I'm just old enough to remember the days when automobile repair depended greatly on the skill and experience of qualified technicians. Now, with the presence of computer chips in nearly all high-tech gadgetry, a mechanic needs sophisticated diagnostic machinery to locate the cause of my car's woes. I don't think that my mechanic is *listening to my engine* like the specialists of the past. Doctors have evolved much the same way. They no longer listen to the patient. Let's be honest, **you** may be a better diagnostician than the doctor you pay to see!

## Kinesiology Evaluation

This is a skillset that takes years to develop and is NOT recognized by the medical profession as a legal approach to diagnose anything. I think that is a good thing as I want as little to do with the standard medical approaches as possible.

I do not diagnose, do not practice under my state license, do not practice medicine, and do not practice to the public. Under my **Pastoral Medical License**, I assist members in a Biblical approach to wellness. This is one reason why I write books, blogs, and newsletters. I still think that we have the right to free speech in this country and that allows me to state my opinion regardless of what the pharmaceutical companies dictate.

So stated, I believe that there are better, more accurate ways to come to a conclusion that someone may wish to treat their symptoms as if they are struggling with Chronic Lyme Disease. Kinesiology, properly applied, is a tool that may point people in the right direction.

## Need a Consultation?

I personally offer what we call a Case Review. We do these over the phone, even if you are local to our clinic. At this writing, our fee is $199 for approximately 30 minutes and I will help you choose a path that's best for you. *However*, our clinic is primarily caring for cancer patients and has a limited availability. Finding a Lyme-literate doctor who is local to you may be your best option.

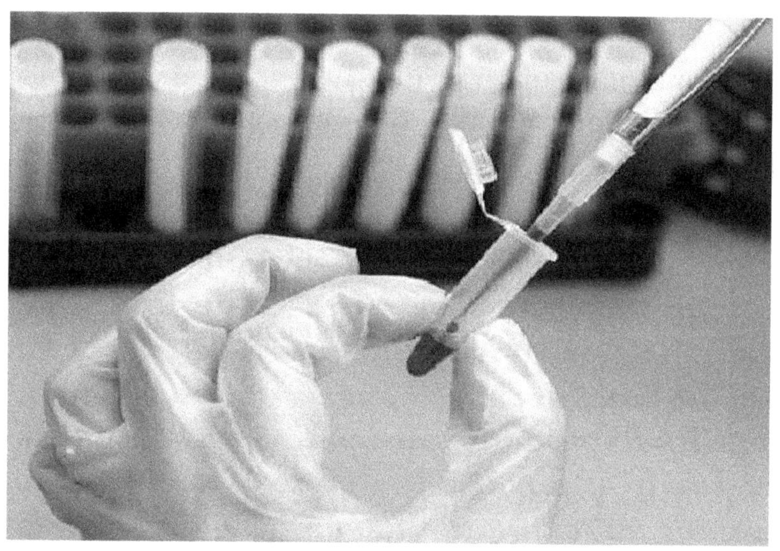

# More Advanced Information: Understanding the Immune Response

*"When wealth is lost, nothing is lost; when health is lost, something is lost; when character is lost, all is lost."*
*-Billy Graham*

## What is Autoimmune Lyme?

Once you've missed the *window of opportunity* of killing the pathogen with an antibiotic, things turn south. Phase 3 Lyme Disease is, after all, what this book is supposed to be about, so what can you do?

81

First, you must remember that Phase 3 Lyme is an autoimmune disorder. Thus, it is necessary to begin with an understanding of what an autoimmune disease really is.

***It is important to understand that an autoimmune disease is a state that the immune system is in. It is not a disease of an organ; and even though it is given a multitude of names depending on the tissue currently affected, it is a state of the immune system attacking the tissue it was meant to protect.***

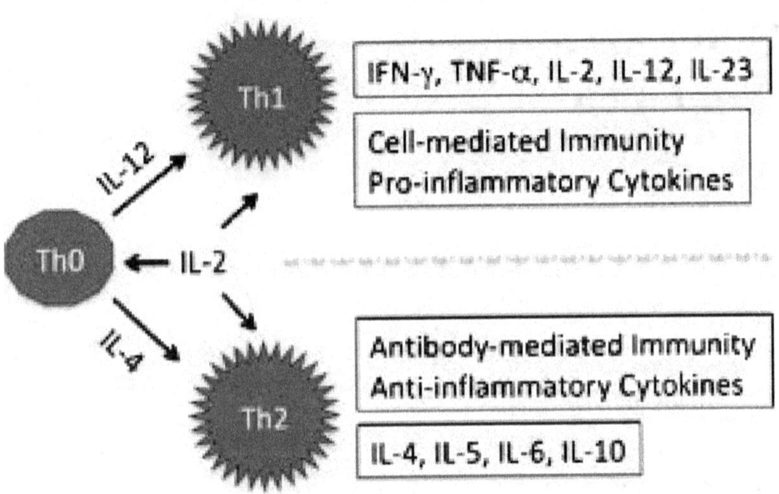


Some highlight points to know about your immune system:

- Your immune system does one thing and only one thing – it **kills** things.

- Your immune system may be separated into two responses – Th1 and Th2 (simplistically, there are more but we'll leave it at that for now)

- Your immune system is supposed to only *turn on* against bio-toxins (living organisms like bacteria, virus, parasites…that is, things that it can kill)

- The Th1 response is the immediate, killer cell response (think of it as the Marine Corps) against the enemy and is the primary killer of antigens like Lyme pathogens and its co-infections. What it *turns on* against is called an *antigen* in the immune response.

- The Th2 response is sent out secondarily and is mainly responsible for making *antibodies* against the *antigen* that the Th1 system *turned on* against. The antibodies *tag* the *antigens* and the Th1 system can then more easily find and kill them.

- Your immune system assists in the cleaning up of old cells necessary for cancer to **not** develop in the first place. This is primarily a Th1 function.

- Both Th1 and Th2 responses are named such because they carry a slurry of different chemicals (immune cells, chemokines, and cytokines) that make up such a response.

An *autoimmune disorder* happens when your immune system starts attacking self-tissue. Really, an autoimmune disease develops because your immune system has *turned-on* against something it found lodged in self-tissue and is now destroying self-tissue as well.

Let's expand that definition a little more so you can fully understand it: If my immune system fires a response against a flu virus I just picked up and it's a particularly virulent virus, a strong Th1 response is released in an attempt to kill the foreign invader and bring me back to health. My "strong Th1 response" is really a collection of different cells that are looking for a battle; they are seeking an enemy with guns loaded. Let's say they find the flu virus and recognize that it is the enemy they were commissioned to kill, they attack it, kill it, and then retreat in victory. The Th1/Th2 system goes back into balance and life is good.

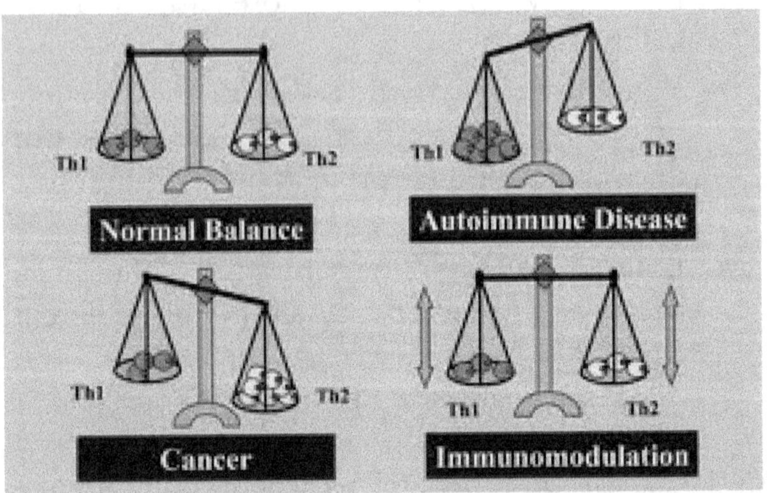

An autoimmune disease begins when, for a multitude of reasons we won't discuss here, stray cytokines from a Th1 response didn't recognize the flu virus as the enemy but recognized something that they were never supposed to recognize as an enemy – let's say a heavy metal toxicity in my thyroid.

Because I was exposed to a great amount of mercury from amalgams, vaccinations, and just living in a toxic world, mercury had lodged in the fat cells surrounding my thyroid and other tissues. My liver, unable to clear out that which I was exposed to, caused my system to shunt the toxicity to fat storage cells for safe keeping. Never was my immune system supposed to *turn-on* against such chemical toxicity!

Is my immune system ever going to be able to kill mercury? Of course not; mercury is an element on the periodic table, not a living organism. If my immune system inadvertently *turns-on* against something that *cannot or will not die*, there will be a lot of collateral damage and I might even begin to start making antibodies against the tissues surrounding the attack. This is an autoimmune disease; it isn't really a disease at all, it is an immune attack on self-tissue because my immune system is firing against something it never should have fired against! Remember, when the immune system *turns-on* against something, it does so until it achieves victory; until it kills it.

In the case of Lyme Disease, in its acute state it is theoretically *killable* by one's immune system. Because it is very virulent, it may take your un-aided immune response some time to make a dent in it. This is a problem because after an indiscriminate amount of time (from a matter of a few days to several weeks), Lyme Disease morphs into its spirochete (viral-like) phase and can move intracellular (within the cell).

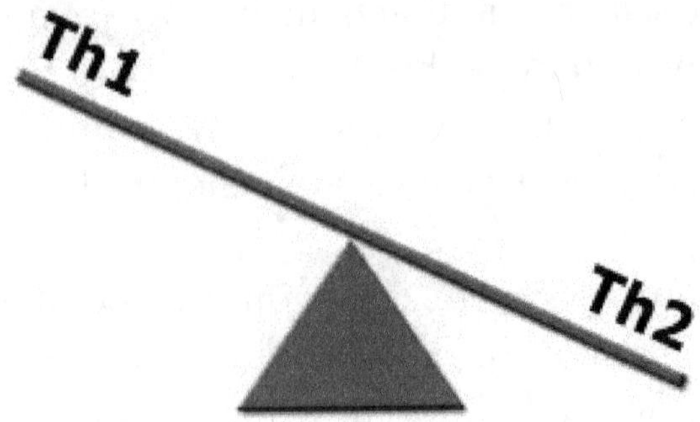


Normally, when a virus attempts to hide from one's immune response by infiltrating a cell, the cell gives off a marker on the outside of the cell membrane to alert the immune cytokines that it has been breached. Immune killer cells then engulf the entire cell, killing both the cell and the invading pathogen and protecting the whole in the process.

However, there are certain bacterial and viral organisms (Lyme being one of these) that have the ability to disarm the cell by disabling the marker that informs the immune system that it has been attacked. I like to describe it this way: Think of a bank robber entering a bank and demanding the teller to fill up his bag with money. The teller pushes a secret button under the counter that summons the police and the thief is apprehended. But a smart thief (Lyme) cut the phone line outside of the building before entering the bank and the secret button does nothing to inform the police car that passes by completely unaware. Tricky little beastie, isn't he?

**Summary**: An autoimmune disease is when your immune system is firing against something (either predominantly Th1 dominant or predominantly Th2 dominant) that it found lodged in self-tissue that either cannot or will not die (as in Lyme) and is destroying self-tissue in the process.

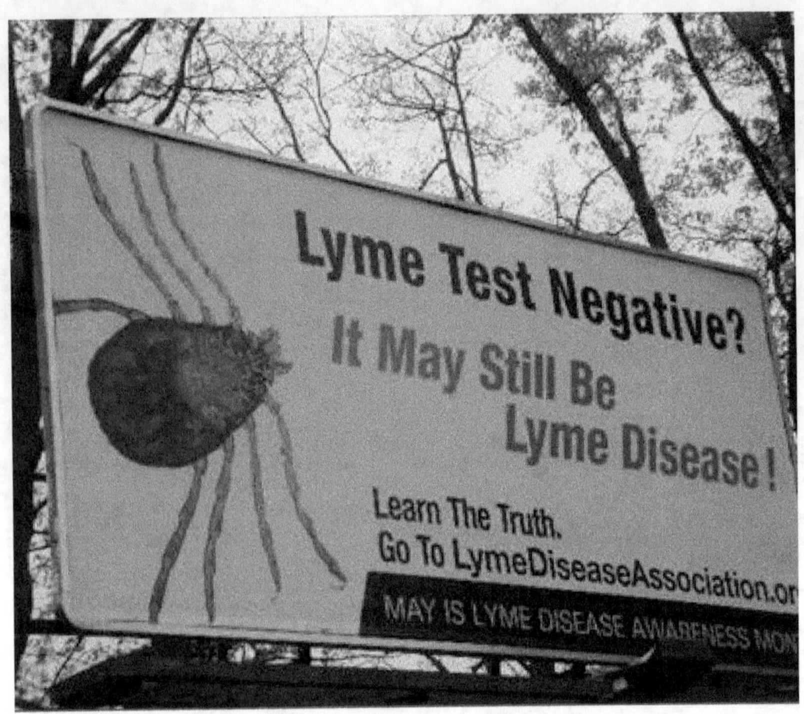


So, what is the **cause** of an autoimmune attack? It's not so much an "immune system gone wrong" as it is an immune system thinking it is doing "right" but firing against something that it can never kill. The only way to ultimately correct an autoimmune disorder is to remove the antigen that it is making war against.

This way you are essentially fooling your immune system to think that it has won, and the enemy is dead. In the case of autoimmune disease against a specific organ like Hashimoto's hypothyroidism, there is little help in direct organ support without correcting the cause. The mechanism for the issue is the immune response in the first place and not that the organ is deficient in any type of nutrient; the reason the person may need hormone replacement (such as Synthroid) in hypothyroidism is because the immune system is actually destroying the cells, but replacement without halting the destruction is missing the point.

## What does this all have to do with Lyme?

What does this all have to do with Lyme? Everything! Remember, Chronic Lyme Disease (CLD) is when the acute infection has moved into a viral-like, spirochete phase that is nearly impossible to kill as it hides inside cells and evades the immune response. When Th1 cytokines cannot find the pathogen, they start to kill surrounding tissue creating an autoimmune disorder.

## How does it progress?

Usually people with Phase 3 Lyme, involving much destruction and therefore many symptoms, have a Th1 dominant autoimmune response; that is, the immune response is stuck in a Th1 (killer cell, Marine Corps) attack. This typically brings about much tissue damage, much inflammation, and a greater number of symptoms that causes them to seek medical care and hopefully arrive at a diagnosis. They often are misdiagnosed as having MS, RA, Hashimoto's, etc. Actually, it may not be a misdiagnosis as all autoimmune disorders have an antigen at its core and that antigen might just be Lyme!

Neither the standard medical nor an alternative healthcare has adequately dealt with autoimmune conditions, including CLD, because most fail to understand the Th1/Th2 issue. Medically, the patient is given long-term antibiotics, anti-malarial drugs, steroids, anti-inflammatories and more that may temporarily relieve the symptoms but do nothing to remove the cause; alternative doctors have supported the organs with glandulars and tried to kill the CLD with herbs or other supplements. Let's face it, if either traditional medical or the alternative models had any great percentage of success treating CLD autoimmune disorder, you wouldn't be reading this book because you probably wouldn't have any symptoms.

It is important to understand that an autoimmune disease is a *state* that the immune system is in. It is *not* a disease of an organ; and even though it is given a multitude of names depending on the tissue currently affected, it is a *state* of the immune system attacking the tissue it was meant to protect.

It's absolutely necessary to figure out if a person is Th1 or Th2 dominant because it will dictate what type of protocols that will be most effective for dampening their immune activity. We know that typical "immune stimulants" like Astragalus, Cats Claw, Samento, Echinacea, Garlic, Glycyrrhizin, Melissa Officinalis, and Maitake mushrooms seem to stimulate a Th1 response. We also know that things like pine bark extract, grape seed extract, green tea extract, Pycnogenol, Resveratrol, and caffeine are things that stimulate the Th2 response. So, if a patient's CLD attack of their joints, brain, muscles, or fatigue is a Th1 dominant response, adding Th1 stimulants will ***make them worse***! You can effectively aid in balancing a Th1 dominant individual by giving Th2 stimulants, and vice versa.

## Custom Formulated Solutions

We have developed and formulated (using specific, researched ingredients) products for all 3 Phases of Lyme. I'll share details on these later, but mention them here:

**Acute LX** – This unique formulation contains berberine, an alkaloid compound found in the roots, rhizomes, stems and bark of several plants commonly used in botanical and Chinese medicine. Berberine has long been recognized as an antimicrobial, antiviral, and anti-parasitic compound. This formulation also includes Cat's claw. This powerful herb has been used for thousands of years for medicinal purposes, which include anti-inflammatory and antiviral effects, as

91

well as stimulation of the immune system. Maitake and Reishi medicinal mushroom extracts are excellent immune system complements that encourage T-Cell and Macrophage attack on invaders. Find it on our store at **shop.ConnersClinic.com/acuteLX**

**Chronic LX** – This has been specially designed for those with chronic, stubborn, and often hidden infections. Artemisia is an excellent fighter of intracellular bacteria as it readily absorbs and passes through cell membranes. Coriolus is one of the best sources of polysaccharides that help stimulate Macrophage attack on co-infections and Monolaurin is a proven, broad-spectrum killer of both gram-positive and gram-negative bacteria. The unique addition of thymus gland tissue gently supports your own production of immune cells. The Sodium Alginate serves as an excellent chelator of lipopolysaccharides, the byproducts of killing bacteria and the unique enzyme blend helps breakdown the bacteria's protective biofilm. Chronic LX would also be a great supplement for other chronic viral, mold, and fungal infections. Find it on our store at **shop.ConnersClinic.com/chronicLX**

**AI** – AI is specially formulated to help rid the body of mold, fungal, Lyme, and other bacteria along with their co-infections without stimulating a strong immune response. Grapeseed extract may serve as a direct attack on pathogens, coupled with the

Glycine, and N-Acetyl Cysteine supporting cellular glutathione production, a key to your own defense. The Phosphatidylcholine and Gamma-tocotrienol support both cell membrane health and, along with Artichoke Leaf Extract, helps with Phase 2.5 and Phase 3 detoxification. The unique enzyme blend is added to for biofilms and Sodium Alginate for a gentle chelation and gut support. Find it on our store at **shop.ConnersClinic.com/ai**

It is often the case that your history will be obvious as to which dominance you are *stuck* in. If you've attempted taking high amounts of Cats Claw, Garlic, and Echinacea in the past only to feel horribly worse afterward, there's a pretty good chance you are Th1 dominant autoimmune. If drinking green tea or coffee takes away your major symptoms, the possibility exists that you are Th1 dominant; if it made you feel worse, you may be Th2 dominant. But do *not* rely on this; it is always wise to do the testing! I wish it were always that easy to detect dominance. Many people just don't seem to get better after giving full effort with numerous nutritional or standard approaches. This should be at least a clue that there is something deeper not being addressed.

Also, you have to be very careful stimulating a Th1 or Th2 response. People can't figure out why they still feel terrible even while taking the boatload of vitamins their nutritionist recommended. If you are stimulating the dominant, hyper-firing system, you are literally throwing fuel on the fire. Autoimmune patients *cannot* take supplements that have both Th1 and Th2 stimulants. You are helping the immune system destroy your body! Do the testing!

## Th1 and Th2 Balancing

There are 2 parts of your immune system: the Th1 and Th2 response. When a person is autoimmune, one of these systems is *hyper-firing* or *dominant*. Balancing this system goes far in reducing a patient's symptoms.

*These Should be Balanced!*

There are specific dietary changes and supplements that can *help* and *hinder* the above response.

*Note: All AI cases need Vitamin D, Glutathione, and Omega 3 fish oils*

94

## Things that Stimulate a Th1 Response

You can take these if you are in Acute (Phase 1) or Chronic (Phase 2) Lyme – note: if taking any of these makes you **worse**, that's a good indication that you are in Phase 3!

- Cats Claw
- Samento
- Echinacea
- Golden Seal
- Red Clover
- Pau D'Arco
- Wild Bergamot (Monarda fistulosa)
- Oregon Grape (Mahonia aquifolium)
- Andrographis (Andrographis paniculata)
- Lignan-vitae (Guaiacum officinale)
- Garlic
- Vitamin C
- Licorice root (Glycyrrhizin)
- Astragalus
- Most Medicinal mushrooms
- Most Chinese Herbs
- All "Immune Stimulants"
- Beta-glucan mushroom
- Maitake mushroom (Grifola frondosa)
- Lemon Balm (Melissa officinalis)

**Things that Stimulate the Th2 Response**

You can take these if you are in Phase 3 Lyme.

- Caffeine (don't add this as this does a number on your adrenals)
- Green Tea
- Grape Seed Extract
- Herbal barks (Cramp Bark, Pine Bark, and White Willow Bark)
- Lycopene
- Resveratrol
- Pycnogenol

This is in no way a complete list, and individuals may react differently than expected!!

Therefore, if a patient is Phase 3 Autoimmune, they should **avoid** Th1 Stimulants and **may** take Th2 Stimulants.


# Treating Acute, Phase 1 Lyme

Definitions Reminder – When the bacteria and/or co-infections are still confined to the blood and extracellular spaces (outside the cells), you are still in Phase 1. The moment one bacterium traverses a cell membrane to enter the *inside* of the cell, we define this as Chronic, Phase 2 Lyme. Once the immune system, in its attempt to kill the pathogen, begins to make antibodies against your own tissues, you are in the Autoimmune, Phase 3.

## Initial, Acute, Bacterial Phase 1

Symptoms of early localized Lyme Disease (Phase 1) begin days or weeks after infection. They are similar to the flu and may include:

- Body-wide itching
- Chills
- Fever
- General ill-feeling
- Headache
- Light-headedness or fainting
- Muscle pain
- Stiff neck

There may be a *bull's eye* rash, a flat or slightly raised red spot at the site of the tick bite but this is often missing or undetectable (especially if the bite is on the head under the cover of hair). If the rash is present, often there is a clear area in the center. It can be small to quite large and look like a red blotch or a traditional bullseye. If what I just said is confusing, well, it is. The initial bite can be confusing and is very often missed with the tick never to be found.

Most commonly, no rash will be detected, and no tick found, and the patient may never experience

97

any of the above *acute phase* symptoms. This is most unfortunate as the patient is destined to move into Phase 2 as no care is received.

Again, if the person is bit in the head, the rash can hide under the hair and never be detected. Some people have a rash that lasts a few hours; others never see a rash and mistakenly attribute their symptoms to a flu or food poisoning.

My rule of thumb: If you live in a Lyme area and get flu-like symptoms during tick season, *treat it as if it is Lyme* and get an antibiotic!!! If you wait for the tests to come back, it may be too late. Find a qualified Lyme-literate MD and get a prescription.

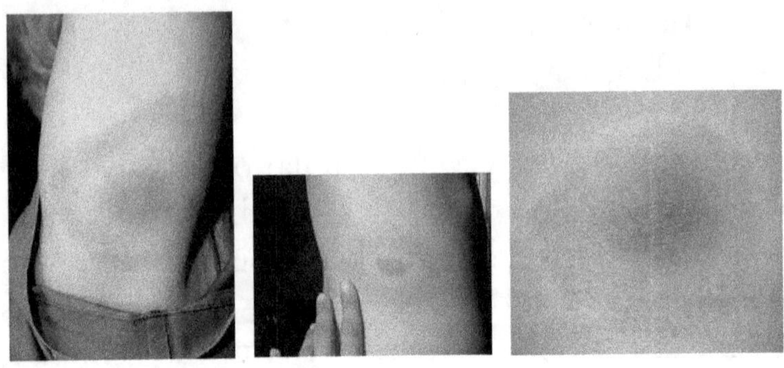

## Treatment Options in Phase 1, Acute Lyme

### Antibiotics

There are four types of antibiotics generally prescribed for Lyme treatment that I'd like to discuss. I am not an MD and cannot write a prescription, so I'll quote Joseph J. Burrascano, M.D., *Board Member, International Lyme and Associated Diseases Society* from his 2008 work entitled *Advanced Topics in Lyme Disease*:

1. "The TETRACYCLINES, including doxycycline and minocycline, are bacteriostatic unless given in high doses. If high blood levels are not attained, treatment failures in early and late disease are common. However, these high doses can be difficult to tolerate. For example, doxycycline can be very effective but only if adequate blood levels are achieved either by high oral doses (300 to 600 mg daily) or by parenteral administration (through an IV). Kill kinetics indicate that a large spike in blood and tissue levels is more effective than sustained levels, which is why with doxycycline, oral doses of 200 mg bid (twice per day) is more effective than 100 mg qid (four doses per day). Likewise, this is why IV doses of 400 mg once a day is more effective than any oral regimen. (I realize IV dosing is not realistic for most patients, see below)

2. PENICILLINS are bactericidal. As would be expected in managing an infection with a gram-negative organism such as Bb, amoxicillin has been shown to be more

effective than oral penicillin V. With cell wall agents such as the penicillins, kill kinetics indicate that sustained bactericidal levels are needed for 72 hours to be effective. Thus, the goal is to try to achieve sustained blood and tissue levels. However, since blood levels are extremely variable among patients, peak and trough levels should be measured (for details, refer to the antibiotic dosage table). Because of its short half-life and need for high levels, amoxicillin is usually administered along with probenecid. An extended release formulation of amoxicillin+clavulanate ("Augmentin XR") may also be considered if adequate trough levels are difficult to attain. An attractive alternative is benzathine penicillin ("Bicillin-LA"- see below). This is an intramuscular depot injection, and although doses are relatively small, the sustained blood and tissue levels are what make this preparation so effective.

3. CEPHALOSPORINS must be of advanced generation: first generation drugs are rarely effective and second-generation drugs are comparable to amoxicillin and doxycycline both in-vitro and in-vivo. Third generation agents are currently the most effective of the cephalosporins because of their very low MBC's (0.06 for ceftriaxone), and relatively long half-life. Cephalosporins have been shown to be effective in penicillin and tetracycline failures. Cefuroxime axetil

(Ceftin), a second-generation agent, is also effective against staph and thus is useful in treating atypical erythema migrans that may represent a mixed infection that contains some of the more common skin pathogens in addition to Bb. Because this agent's G.I. side effects and high cost, it is not often used as first line drug. As with the penicillins, try to achieve high, sustained blood and tissue levels by frequent dosing and/or the use of probenecid. Measure peak and trough blood levels when possible. When choosing a third-generation cephalosporin, there are several points to remember: Ceftriaxone is administered twice daily (an advantage for home therapy) but has 95% biliary excretion and can crystallize in the biliary tree with resultant colic and possible cholecystitis. GI excretion results in a large impact on gut flora. Biliary and superinfection problems with ceftriaxone can be lessened if this drug is given in interrupted courses (known commonly as *pulse therapy* - refer to chapter on this on page 20 of Dr. Burrascano's book for more info on this), so the current recommendation is to administer it four days in a row each week. Cefotaxime, which must be given at least every eight hours or as a continuous infusion, is less convenient, but as it has only 5% biliary excretion, it never causes biliary concretions, and may have less impact on gut flora.

4. RYTHROMYCIN has been shown to be almost ineffective as monotherapy. The azalide azithromycin is somewhat more effective but only minimally so when given orally. As an IV drug, much better results are seen. Clarithromycin is more effective as an oral agent than azithromycin but can be difficult to tolerate due to its tendency to promote yeast overgrowth, bad aftertaste, and poor GI tolerance at the high doses needed. These problems are much less severe with the ketolide telithromycin, which is generally well tolerated. Erythromycins (and the advanced generation derivatives mentioned above) have impressively low MBCs and they do concentrate in tissues and penetrate cells, so they theoretically should be ideal agents. So why is it that erythromycin ineffective, and why have initial clinical results with azithromycin (and to a lesser degree, clarithromycin) have been disappointing? It has been suggested that when Bb is within a cell, it is held within a vacuole and bathed in fluid of low pH, and this acidity may inactivate azithromycin and clarithromycin. Therefore, they are administered concurrently with hydroxychloroquine or amantadine, which raise vacuolar pH, rendering these antibiotics more effective. It is not known whether this same technique will make erythromycin a more effective antibiotic in LB. Another alternative is to administer

azithromycin parenterally. Results are excellent but expect to see abrupt Jarisch-Herxheimer reactions.

### Real World Uses

Again, if you even *think* that you have an Acute Lyme infection, antibiotics are the way to go. I also suggest *adding* alternative herbs and vitamins at this stage to help the immune system respond. This is where our **Acute LX** comes in, adding to an antibiotic approach.

In my three experiences with Acute Lyme, I took amoxicillin with exceptional results. However, my first incidence was easy to spot with a bulls-eye rash that appeared painted upon my belly and severe flu-like symptoms. One day of 500mg amoxicillin, taken twice daily, knocked out all of my symptoms. I only completed 3 days of antibiotics though I'd never suggest anyone to follow my lead on that. The next Lyme episode went undiagnosed for nearly 5 days as I had no rash and very little exposure to the outside. At first, I thought that I had food poisoning, then the flu. After 4 days I finally tested myself Kinesiologically and sure enough, it was Lyme. Amoxicillin saved the day again.

Everyone is different, and for many, doxycycline is the therapy of choice for Acute Lyme. It is my opinion that messing around with any other therapy to kill Acute Lyme is like playing with fire. Don't do it.

## Acute LX

I formulated **Acute LX** specifically for Lyme Phase 1. It can also be used to treat any acute infection. The ingredients are well researched:

This unique formulation contains berberine, an alkaloid compound found in the roots, rhizomes, stems and bark of several plants commonly used in botanical and Chinese medicine. Berberine has long been recognized as an antimicrobial, antiviral, and anti-parasitic compound. This formulation also includes Cat's claw. This powerful herb has been used for thousands of years for medicinal purposes, which include anti-inflammatory and antiviral effects, as well as stimulation of the immune system. Maitake and Reishi medicinal mushroom extracts are excellent immune system complements that encourage T-Cell and Macrophage attack on invaders.

Acute LX is targeted nutrition for those concerned about contracting a biotoxin and those that feel they may have been acutely exposed. Although especially designed for bacteria, would also be a great supplement for other acute viral, mold and fungal infections.

## *Ingredients*

**Berberine (Berberis vulgaris)**: Berberine has demonstrated significant activity against a wide variety of organisms including a broad spectrum of bacteria, yeasts, fungus and parasites. Its mechanism of action is thought to result in part from its characteristic structure, which is that of a planar cationic molecule. This structural arrangement enables it to intercalate the DNA structure.[30]

**Cat's Claw (Uncaria tomentosa)**: Cat's Claw, also known as the "life-giving vine of Peru," "saventaro," or "uña de gato," is indigenous to the Amazon rain forest and other tropical areas of South and Central America.[31] Its alkaloids are purported to exhibit various pharmacologic activities, including anti-inflammatory, antiviral, antioxidant, immune-stimulating, anti-rheumatic, and antineoplastic properties.[32] [33] It has been reported to possibly benefit those with autoimmune arthritis as well.[34]

---

[30] Jennings BR, Ridler PJ. Interaction of chromosomal stains with DNA. An electrofluorescence study. Biophys Struct Mech. 1983;10(1-2):71-9

[31] Altitudinal variation of berberine, total phenolics and flavanoid content in Thalictrum foliolosum and their correlation with antimicrobial and antioxidant activities. Journal of Ayurveda and Integrative Medicine, 9(3), 169-176. Doi: 0.1016/j. jaim.2017.02.010

[32] Zhang, D., Ke, L., Ni, Z., Chen, Y., Zhang, L. H., Zhu, S. H., ... Shi, Y. Q. (2017). Berberine containing quadruple therapy for initial Helicobacter pylori eradication: An open-label randomized phase IV trial. Medicine, 96(32). doi:10.1097/MD.0000000000007697

[33] Keplinger K, Laus G, Wurm M et al. Uncaria tomentosa (Willd.) DC. Ethno-medicinal use and new pharmacological, toxicological and botanical results. J Ethnopharmaco, 1999; 64:23–34

**Maitake and Reishi Mushroom extracts (Grifola frondosa and Ganoderma lucidum)**: Mushroom polysaccharides elicit an immune-modulatory response with impact on the expression of cytokines IL-1α, IL-6, IL-10 and TNF-α in human macrophages with and without LPS stimulation.[35]

We utilize a hot water extraction for the increased antioxidant properties as hot-water extracts show high scavenging ability on superoxide anions.[36]

## *Directions*

1-2 capsules can be taken three times per day with or without food.

Find **Acute LX** on our store at
**shop.ConnersClinic.com/acuteLX**

---

[34] Herbal medicines: a guide for health-care professionals. http://hhmicromedex01:81/hcs/librarian/PFPUI/2dleUVoy2UKCTRA

[35] National Center for Complementary and Alternative Medicines. Herbs at a glance. Cat's claw. http://nccam.nih.gov/health/cat- claw/#uses

[36] Dudics S, Langan D, Meka RR, et al. Natural Products for the Treatment of Autoimmune Arthritis: Their Mechanisms of Action, Targeted Delivery, and Interplay with the Host Microbiome. Int J Mol Sci. 2018;19(9):2508. Published 2018 Aug 24. doi:10.3390/ijms19092508

# Treating Chronic, Phase 2 Lyme

Definitions Reminder – When the bacteria and/or co-infections are still confined to the blood and extracellular spaces (outside the cells), you are still in Phase 1. The moment one bacterium traverses a cell membrane to enter the *inside* of the cell, we define this as Chronic, Phase 2 Lyme. Once the immune system, in its attempt to kill the pathogen, begins to make antibodies against your own tissues, you are in the Autoimmune, Phase 3.

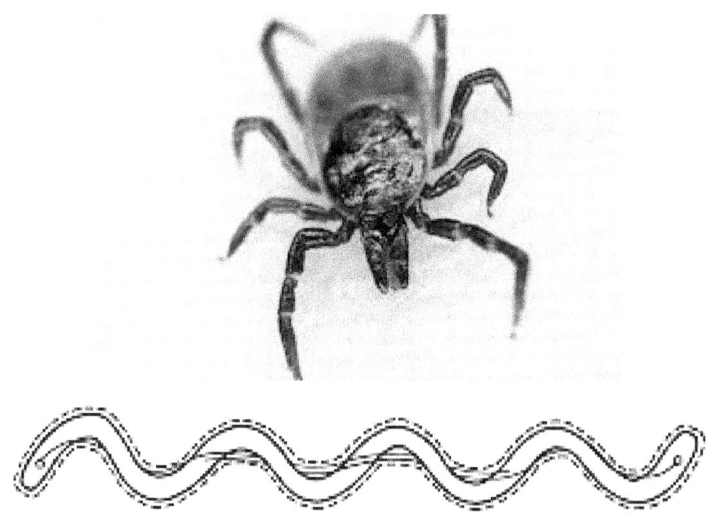

Schematic representation of a spirochete

Again, the autoimmune response is an inflammatory response, which produces chemicals called cytokines, which are part of the body's natural defense system against outside invaders. Remember, the body's immune system may be separated into a Th1 and a Th2 response. The Th1 response may be thought of as the police force or Marine Corps, the body's initial strike force against an invader or what is called an antigen.

In a *perfect world*, when an antigen (in this case Lyme and its co-infections) is present, the Th1 system (the *killer* side of the immune system) fires to try to kill the infection; since the bug happens to be of a nasty persuasion and strong enough to resist the Th1 response, soon (usually within 24-48 hours) the Th2 system kicks in, creates antibodies against the Lyme, tagging them, so that appropriate Th1 white blood cells (killer cells) can finish them off. In *reality*, this rarely happens with Lyme. The Th1 response is *not* strong enough to kill the Lyme pathogens and they morph into a viral-like state and go intracellular to hide from the immune response. Your Th2 cytokines start producing antibodies to the tissues it searched in and you are in for a world of trouble because we *passed directly to the autoimmune phase*!

## Timeline

It may take weeks or years for your body (your immune system) to begin making antibodies to self-tissue. A person can be in Phase 1 for a matter of days before the infection moves intracellular, but it usually takes weeks to months before this occurs.

**Example:**

April 1<sup>st</sup> – You notice a spot on your leg while working outside. You ignore it until you come inside later and see that the spot has reddened and increased in size to about the diameter of a quarter. Looking closer, you notice a black speck in the center. Being literate about the possibility of Lyme Disease, you remove the speck and examine it with a magnifying glass to become shocked that it actually is a tiny tick. You decide (maybe foolishly) to wait to see if any symptoms appear before doing anything else.

April 3<sup>rd</sup> – You begin to feel stomach upset and general malaise. You forgot about the tick bite and blame the sick feeling on the dinner you ate at the greasy spoon restaurant last night that you knew you shouldn't have ordered. The day progresses with more symptoms and worsening issues.

April 4<sup>th</sup> – Your spouse and children never got sick from eating at the same restaurant and you begin to question your diagnosis. Towards evening, as your symptoms don't abate, you recall your tick bite and begin the put the pieces together.
April 5<sup>th</sup> – You call your primary physician and schedule an appointment but, since it's now Friday, they can't get you in until Wednesday the following week. You tell yourself you'll be okay until then.

April 6<sup>th</sup> – You wake Saturday morning vomiting and extremely sick. Your intestines feel like someone is kicking you with steel-toed boots. Your spouse convinces you to go to the emergency room and drives there as soon as possible. Unfortunately, after 3 hours in your small rural hospital, after blood tests come back normal, they tell you that you probably have either a stomach bug or food poisoning and then release you with anti-nausea meds. No antibiotics were prescribed as the doctor doesn't believe in Lyme Disease.

April 7th-9th – Your symptoms wax and wane over the next several days with the help of the medications and you finally get to go and see your primary doctor.

April 10th – At your visit to your primary doctor, she listened to your history and agrees that Lyme Disease may be a possibility. But, since she is fairly young and believes in objective testing, she refuses to make a clinical diagnosis without running labs to confirm. She orders a Western blot test and tells you that she'll have the office staff call you when the results come in. You leave.

April 10th – April 15th – Your symptoms continue to wax and wane and you continue to use OTC medications as well as the prescriptions.

April 15th – You get a call from the doctor's office telling you that your Western blot test came back negative so, "You don't have Lyme." You are confused but relieved.

April 15<sup>th</sup>-the next several months – You have days when you have little to no symptoms and days of extreme fatigue and weird pain that is difficult to describe. Your coworkers joke that you're just getting older and you begin to question food allergies or maybe the beginning of arthritis.

August 15<sup>th</sup> – You've returned to your primary doctor after much consideration and, after listening to your plight, she orders a full blood work-up and thorough examination. To your dismay and relief, everything is normal. She suggests that stress is probably at play and you recall that events over the past several months have been unusually burdensome with the death of your father-in-law, though it wasn't a surprise, he was 93. But, you rationalize, loss is loss and maybe that's what is going on.

From August through next April, your general well-being has been on a general decline. You still have days of relative normalcy but overall, you have forgotten how normal really feels. After the advice of your doctor, you've begun to see a therapist.

**Does this sound like a timeline that's remotely familiar to you? There can be hundreds of variations with many scenarios ending far worse! In general, the Lyme infection has continued to progress throughout the time, and we can recap the same story with how the infection behaved:**

April 1$^{st}$ – You notice a spot on your leg while working outside. You ignore it until you come inside later and see that the spot has reddened and increased in size to about the diameter of a quarter. Looking closer, you notice a black speck in the center. Being literate about the possibility of Lyme Disease, you remove the speck and examine it with a magnifying glass to become shocked that it actually is a tiny tick. You decide (maybe foolishly) to wait to see if any symptoms appear before doing anything else. ***When you were bit by the tick, it injected Borellia and certain co-infections into your blood that began to circulate and attempt to use your body as a host to reproduce and raise a family.***

April 3$^{rd}$ – You begin to feel stomach upset and general malaise. You forgot about the tick bite and blame the sick feeling on the dinner you ate at the greasy spoon restaurant last night that you knew you shouldn't have ordered. The day progresses with more symptoms and worsening issues. ***The bacteria and viruses are continuing to reproduce and surge throughout your body. If you did have some antibiotics at home, taking them may have immediately destroyed the majority of pathogens and your immune system.***

April 4$^{th}$ – Your spouse and children never got sick from eating at the same restaurant and you begin to question your diagnosis. Towards evening, as your symptoms don't abate, you recall your tick bite and begin the put the pieces together.

April 5th – You call your primary physician and schedule an appointment but, since it's now Friday, they can't get you in until Wednesday the following week. You tell yourself you'll be okay until then. ***The longer you wait to receive care, whether an antibiotic to kill the bacteria or immune support to help your own system kill the infection, the greater chance the pathogens will leave the blood, enter the extracellular spaces, and then eventually enter the cells.***

April 6th – You wake Saturday morning vomiting and extremely sick. Your intestines feel like someone is kicking you with steel-toed boots. Your spouse convinces you to go to the emergency room and drives there as soon as possible. Unfortunately, after 3 hours in your small rural hospital, after blood tests come back normal, they tell you that you probably have either a stomach bug or food poisoning and then release you with anti-nausea meds. No antibiotics were prescribed as the doctor doesn't believe in Lyme Disease.

April 7th-9th – Your symptoms wax and wane over the next several days with the help of the medications and you finally get to go and see your primary doctor.

April 10th – At your visit to your primary doctor, she listened to your history and agrees that Lyme

Disease may be a possibility. But, since she is fairly young and believes in objective testing, she refuses to make a clinical diagnosis without running labs to confirm. She orders a Western blot test and tells you that she'll have the office staff call you when the results come in. You leave. *As your disease continues, failure to make a clinical decision based on signs and symptoms allows the infection to grow unabated. Relying on a Western blot, with its 35% accuracy, is poor practice at best. While I find it laughable that doctors tend to give out antibiotics like candy for childhood ear infections and sore throats, they turn into a miser when someone hints of Lyme Disease.*

April 10th –April 15th – Your symptoms continue to wax and wane and you continue to use OTC medications as well as the prescriptions.

April 15th – You get a call from the doctor's office telling you that your Western blot test came back negative so, "You don't have Lyme." You are confused but relieved. *While I would hope that a doctor would continue to investigate for a cause, this example rings true for many. They are left unknowing, confused, and sick.*

April 15th-the next several months – You have days when you have little to no symptoms and days of extreme fatigue and weird pain that is difficult to describe. Your coworkers joke that you're just getting older and you begin to question food allergies or maybe the beginning of arthritis. ***Lyme patients find this common as well. The disease is slowly progressing through their body, affecting different systems and giving them a wide range of diverse symptoms that can change from day to day. This is really infuriating to me. Physicians need to make clinical decisions based on signs, symptoms, history, and a little bit of common sense! There is a window of time, often a brief window of time, that effective care with antibiotics help. When this window closes, you are in Phase 2!***

August 15<sup>th</sup> – You've returned to your primary doctor after much consideration and, after listening to your plight, she orders a full blood work-up and thorough examination. To your dismay and relief, everything is normal. She suggests that stress is probably at play and your recall that events over the past several months have been unusually burdensome with the death of your father-in-law, though it wasn't a surprise, he was 93. But, you rationalize, loss is loss and maybe that's what is going on. ***You may have already entered Phase 2 and antibiotics will help temporarily but can only be a piece of the solution if at all. When you missed the window of opportunity to eradicate it with antibiotics, you doomed yourself to a more difficult path.***

115

From August through next April, your general well-being has been on a general decline. You still have days of relative normalcy but overall, you have forgotten how normal really feels. After the advice of your doctor, you've begun to see a therapist. ***At this point you may be in Phase 3, though you are certainly in Phase 2. The brain may be affected, and the range of chronic symptoms can vary across the board. Again, the longer you wait to address the problem, the more progression occurs.***

Note: The major reason *why* the blood tests for Lyme are so highly inaccurate is that the quantities of antibodies are never created for a pathogen the immune system could not detect. Physicians *must* rely on signs, symptoms, history, and a little bit of common sense!

**So again, this is really important:**

Phase 1 and 2 Lyme patients *can* take immune (Th1) stimulants
Phase 3 (Autoimmune) Lyme patients *cannot* take immune (Th1) stimulants

# Treatment Options in Phase 2, Chronic Lyme

## Long-Term Antibiotics

Though I am not a fan of long-term antibiotic therapy, it has helped some people. The collateral damage done to one's microbiota can be horrific in itself. I would much rather do as many natural approaches and use antibiotics sparingly as needed.

## Chronic LX

I developed **Chronic LX** specifically for Phase 2 Lyme. You could do well combining it with the **Acute LX** to give an even better response. It has been scientifically formulated for those with chronic, stubborn, and often hidden infections. Artemisia is an excellent fighter of intracellular bacteria as it readily absorbs and passes through cell membranes. Coriolus is one of the best sources of polysaccharides that help stimulate Macrophage attack on co-infections and Monolaurin is a proven, broad-spectrum killer of both gram-positive and gram-negative bacteria. The unique addition of thymus gland tissue gently supports your own production of immune cells. The Sodium Alginate serves as an excellent chelator of lipopolysaccharides, the byproducts of killing bacteria and the unique enzyme blend helps breakdown the bacteria's protective biofilm. LX Chronic would also be a great supplement for other chronic viral, mold and fungal infections.

## *Ingredients*

**Artemisia annua (sweet wormwood):** Artemisinin, extracted from the medicinal plant Artemisia sp. is an effective anti-malarial drug. In 2015, elucidation of the effectiveness of artemisinin as a potent anti-malarial drug was even acknowledged with a Nobel prize.[37] Recently, it has also been investigated for their antineoplasia properties, with interesting and promising results.[38] Artemisia annua also supports various conditions such as diabetes, heart diseases, arthritis and eczema and possess- es various effects such as antibacterial, antioxidant, anticoccidial, and antiviral effects.[39]

**Thymus Tissue:** Thymus tissue concentrate derived from pure, lyophilized tissue concentrates from New Zealand, which is considered the cleanest

---

[37] Kiani BH, Suberu J, Mirza B. Cellular engineering of Artemisia annua and Artemisia dubia with the rol ABC genes for enhanced production of potent anti-malari- al drug artemisinin. Malar J. 2016;15(1):252. Published 2016 May 4. doi:10.1186/s12936-016-1312-8

[38] Isani G, Bertocchi M, Andreani G, et al. Cytotoxic Effects of Artemisia annua L. and Pure Artemisinin on the D-17 Canine Osteosarcoma Cell Line. Oxid Med Cell Longev. 2019;2019:1615758. Published 2019 Jul 4. doi:10.1155/2019/1615758

[39] Alesaeidi S, Miraj S. A Systematic Review of Anti-malarial Properties, Immunosuppressive Properties, Anti-inflammatory Properties, and Anti-cancer Properties of Artemisia Annua. Electron Physician. 2016;8(10):3150–3155. Published 2016 Oct 25. doi:10.19082/3150

and most environmentally responsible country to source from on the planet.

**Sodium Alginate (Grifola frondosa and Ganoderma lucidum):** Sodium alginate is a soluble dietary fiber extracted from brown seaweed and its solution has been used to support gut healing, bind toxins in the intestinal tract, and as a hemostatic agent to support gastrointestinal bleeding due to gastric ulcers.[40] [41]

**Turkey-tail Mushroom Extract (Coriolus Versicolor):** The polysaccharo-peptide (PSP) isolated from the Coriolus versicolor (Yun zhi) has its effects on various immune subsets, and the positive clinical data has led to its widespread adoption as an adjunct in neoplasias and immune therapies. Ancient Chinese formulations of CV have long been believed to generally promote health, strength, and longevity. Laboratory studies suggest it may have antimicrobial, antiviral, and anti-tumor properties.[42] [43]

---

[40] Horibe S, Tanahashi T, Kawauchi S, Mizuno S, Rikitake Y. Preventative Effects of Sodium Alginate on Indomethacin-induced Small-intestinal Injury in Mice. Int J Med Sci. 2016;13(9):653–663. Published 2016 Aug 1. doi:10.7150/ijms.16232

[41] Mackie AR, Macierzanka A, Aarak K, et al. Sodium alginate decreases the permeability of intestinal mucus. Food Hydrocoll. 2016;52:749–755. doi:10.1016/j.food- hyd.2015.08.004

[42] Saleh MH, Rashedi I, Keating A. Immunomodulatory Properties of Coriolus versicolor: The Role of Polysaccharopeptide. Front Immunol. 2017;8:1087. Published 2017 Sep 6. doi:10.3389/fimmu.2017.01087

[43] Friedman M. Mushroom Polysaccharides: Chemistry and Antiobesity, Antidiabetes, Anticancer, and Antibiotic Properties in Cells, Rodents, and Humans. Foods. 2016;5(4):80. Published 2016 Nov 29.

**Monolaurin (monolaurate):** Monolaurin is a natural compound found in coconut oil and is known for its protective biological activities as an antimicrobial agent. It has also been shown to have antifungal activity against a variety of biofilms as measured by decreased numbers of viable biofilm-associated bacteria as well as decreased biofilm biomass.[44] [45]

**Enzyme blend (Glucoamylase, Chitosanase, Cellulase, Hemicellulase, Pectinase, Beta-Glucanase):** Our unique enzyme formula supports normal gastrointestinal function and microbiota by assisting degradation of biofilm of bacteria and yeast common with chronic infections. It has been shown that enzymes act synergistically, as demonstrated by crystal violet staining of static biofilms, significantly reducing viable cell counts compared to individual enzyme treatment in the dynamic model.[46] The biofilm matrix is the glue that holds cells together and can be key to protect invading species and up to

doi:10.3390/foods5040080

[44] Seleem D, Chen E, Benso B, Pardi V, Murata RM. In vitro evaluation of antifungal activity of monolaurin against Candida albicans biofilms. PeerJ. 2016;4:e2148. Published 2016 Jun 22. doi:10.7717/peerj.2148

[45] Hess DJ, Henry-Stanley MJ, Wells CL. The Natural Surfactant Glycerol Monolaurate Significantly Reduces Development of Staphylococcus aureus and Enterococ- cus faecalis Biofilms. Surg Infect (Larchmt). 2015;16(5):538–542. doi:10.1089/sur.2014.162

[46] Olsen NMC, Thiran E, Hasler T, et al. Synergistic Removal of Static and Dynamic Staphylococcus aureus Biofilms by Combined Treatment with a Bacteriophage Endolysin and a Polysaccharide Depolymerase. Viruses. 2018;10(8):438. Published 2018 Aug 18. doi:10.3390/v10080438

80% of human bacterial infections are biofilm associated.[47] [48]

## *Directions*

Take 2-6 capsules daily, preferably 30 minutes away from food, or as recommended by your Health Care Professional. I recommend combining this with **Acute LX** as well.

Find them on our store at
**shop.ConnersClinic.com/chronicLX** and
**shop.ConnersClinic.com/acuteLX**

# Treating Autoimmune, Phase 3 Lyme

Definitions Reminder – When the bacteria and/or co-infections are still confined to the blood and extracellular spaces (outside the cells), you are still in Phase 1. The moment one bacterium traverses a cell membrane to enter the *inside* of the cell, we define this as Chronic, Phase 2 Lyme. Once the immune

---

[47] Visick KL, Schembri MA, Yildiz F, Ghigo JM. Biofilms 2015: Multidisciplinary Approaches Shed Light into Microbial Life on Surfaces. J Bacteriol. 2016;198(19):2553–2563. Published 2016 Sep 9. doi:10.1128/JB.00156-16
[48] Biofilm infections, their resilience to therapy and innovative treatment strategies. J Intern Med. 2012 Dec;272(6):541-61. doi: 10.1111/joim.12004. Epub 2012 Oct 29

system, in its attempt to kill the pathogen, begins to make antibodies against your own tissues, you are in the Autoimmune, Phase 3.

Refer back to the common example that leads you to develop an autoimmune response. Once a patient has started to create self-antibodies (antibodies to your own tissue), the game changes.

As a physician, if you ignore the Th1/Th2 immune response in treating a patient with Phase 3 Lyme, both the traditional medical and the traditional alternative models of care are doomed to failure. The most important battle to fight is to calm down their immune response and stop the destruction and kill the pathogen through another route!!

The *new model* we are proposing is simply to be more specific. If *your* Autoimmune, Phase 3 Lyme is a hyper-Th1 attack (Th1 dominant) against the antigen and its co-infections, doesn't it make sense to do everything possible to find out how to remove it while calming down the Th1 dominance? I'm no rocket scientist, but this makes sense to me. It's logical and possible to find the specific biochemical pattern perpetrating the response so we can determine how we treat them.

If you can understand this piece and the role of the immune system, you can understand how antigens (non-living toxins or nasty, hard to kill Lyme, virus, mold, candida...) *can* be at the heart of many autoimmune disorders, and even cancer.

A *major* part of my practice is *identifying* and *eliminating* antigens! In doing so, the body can return to homeostasis (balance) and miraculously heal itself!

## Treatment Options in Phase 3, Autoimmune Lyme

### AI

AI has a unique combination of immune (Th1) suppressors/regulators and direct killers.

Remember, once you have self-antibodies, you can no longer use immune stimulators to kill the Lyme. Using immune stimulators at this point will simply help your immune system kill your self-tissue (that which you have antibodies against.)

One indication that you are in Phase 3 is that you react negatively (your symptoms worsen) when you take immune stimulants!

Again, don't take immune stimulants when you believe you are in Phase 3. What *should* you do then? Try our **AI** product:

Are you struggling with symptoms of an autoimmune disorder? The stimulation of an immediate immune response may worsen the clinical condition. In the presence of self-antibodies, an immune stimulation may enhance the attack against self-tissue. Therefore, it may be contraindicative to use immune stimulating nutrition in such cases. This makes it difficult to choose a protocol that will both kill a pathogen and not stimulate or utilize your own immune system to do so.

**AI** is specially formulated to help rid the body of mold, fungal, Lyme and other bacteria along with their co-infections without stimulating a strong immune response. Grapeseed extract may serve as a direct attack on pathogens, coupled with the Glycine, and N-Acetyl Cysteine supporting cellular glutathione production, a key to your own defense. The Phosphatidylcholine and Gamma-tocotrienol support both cell membrane health and, along with Artichoke Leaf Extract, helps with Phase 2.5 and Phase 3 detoxification. The unique enzyme blend is added to for biofilms and Sodium Alginate for a gentle chelation and gut support.

### *Ingredients*

**Gamma-tocotrienol**: Vitamin E tocotrienols are most effective in preventing lipid oxidation and have been highlighted as a superior antioxidant.[49] They

---

[49] Shahidi F, de Camargo AC. Tocopherols and Tocotrienols in Common and Emerging Dietary Sources: Occurrence, Applications, and Health Benefits. Int J Mol Sci. 2016;17(10):1745. Published 2016 Oct 20.

possess potent antioxidant and anti-inflammatory activities and studies show use provides a marked reduction in the severity of histopathological changes observed in autoimmune arthritis.[50]

**Resveratrol**: Many studies have shown that resveratrol has antioxidant, anti-inflammatory, and neuroprotective properties as it suppresses microglia activation, and promotes Th2 responses by increasing anti-inflammatory cytokines, essential for those with autoimmune disorders. It can also promote neurogenesis and prevent hippocampal damage. In addition, the antioxidant activity of resveratrol plays an important role in neuronal differentiation through the activation of silent information regulator-1 (SIRT1).[51] Moreover, resveratrol regulates immunity by interfering with immune cell regulation, proinflammatory cytokines' synthesis, and gene expression.[52]

**Curcumin (C3 Curcuminoids)**: Curcumin has a wide range of beneficial properties e.g. anti-

---

doi:10.3390/ijms17101745

[50] Zainal Z, Rahim AA, Radhakrishnan AK, Chang SK, Khaza'ai H. Investigation of the curative effects of palm vitamin E tocotrienols on autoimmune arthritis disease in vivo. Sci Rep. 2019;9(1):16793. Published 2019 Nov 14. doi:10.1038/s41598-019-53424-7

[51] Gomes BAQ, Silva JPB, Romeiro CFR, et al. Neuroprotective Mechanisms of Resveratrol in Alzheimer's Disease: Role of SIRT1. Oxid Med Cell Longev. 2018;2018:8152373. Published 2018 Oct 30. doi:10.1155/2018/8152373

[52] Malaguarnera L. Influence of Resveratrol on the Immune Response. Nutrients. 2019;11(5):946. Published 2019 Apr 26. doi:10.3390/nu11050946

125

inflammatory, anti-oxidant, anti-cancer, anti-proliferative, anti-fungal and anti-microbial.[53] Its anti-inflammatory mechanism is attributed through inhibition of inducible nitric oxide synthase (iNOS), Cycloxygenase-2 (COX-2), inhibition in production of pro-inflammatory cytokines [IL-1, IL-6, IL-8, IL-12, interferon γ (IFN-γ), tumor necrosis factor-α (TNF-α).

**Grape Seed Extract**: Grape seeds are considered one of the most import- ant sources for phenolic and other compounds that work against biofilm production.[54]

**Sodium Alginate (Grifola frondosa and Ganoderma lucidum)**: Sodium alginate is a soluble dietary fiber extracted from brown seaweed and its solution has been used to support GUT healing, bind toxins in the intestinal tract, and as a hemostatic agent to aid in gastrointestinal bleeding due to gastric ulcers.[55] [56]

---

[53] Hewlings SJ, Kalman DS. Curcumin: A Review of Its' Effects on Human Health. Foods. 2017;6(10):92. Published 2017 Oct 22. doi:10.3390/- foods6100092

[54] Al-Mousawi, A.H., Al-kaabi, S.J., Albaghdadi, A.J.H. et al. Effect of Black Grape Seed Extract (Vitis vinifera) on Biofilm Formation of Methicillin-Resis- tant Staphylococcus aureus and Staphylococcus haemolyticus. Curr Microbiol (2019) doi:10.1007/s00284-019-01827-0

[55] Horibe S, Tanahashi T, Kawauchi S, Mizuno S, Rikitake Y. Preventative Effects of Sodium Alginate on Indomethacin-induced Small-intestinal Injury in Mice. Int J Med Sci. 2016;13(9):653â€"663. Published 2016 Aug 1. doi:10.7150/ijms.16232

[56] Mackie AR, Macierzanka A, Aarak K, et al. Sodium alginate decreases the permeability of intestinal mucus. Food Hydrocoll.

**N-Acetyl L-Cysteine (NAC)**: NAC is widely known as a precursor to the antioxidant glutathione as it modulates glutamatergic, neurotrophic, and inflammatory pathways.[57]

**Glycine**: Glycine acts as precursor for several key metabolites of low molecular weight such as creatine, glutathione, haem, purines, and porphyrins. Supplementation of glycine is effectual in aiding metabolic disorders such as cardiovascular diseases, several inflammatory diseases, obesity, cancers, neurological disorders, and diabetes.[58] Glycine decreases the levels of oxidative stress markers in liver and helps balance glutathione levels leading to reduced oxidative stress.[59]

**Phosphatidylcholine**: Phosphatidylcholine is the major phospholipid in bile, which is the major route for elimination of cholesterol and toxins from the liver. Bile is also the major route of excretion of trace metals, particularly arsenic, copper,

---

2016;52:749â€"755. doi:10.1016/j.foodhyd.2015.08.004

[57] Bavarsad Shahripour R, Harrigan MR, Alexandrov AV. N-acetylcysteine (NAC) in neurological disorders: mechanisms of action and therapeutic opportunities. Brain Behav. 2014;4(2):108â€"122. doi:10.1002/brb3.208

[58] Razak MA, Begum PS, Viswanath B, Rajagopal S. Multifarious Beneficial Effect of Nonessential Amino Acid, Glycine: A Review. Oxid Med Cell Longev. 2017;2017:1716701. doi:10.1155/2017/1716701

[59] El-Hafidi M, Franco M, RamÃrez AR, et al. Glycine Increases Insulin Sensitivity and Glutathione Biosynthesis and Protects against Oxidative Stress in a Model of Sucrose-Induced Insulin Resistance. Oxid Med Cell Longev. 2018;2018:2101562. Published 2018 Feb 21. doi:10.1155/2018/2101562

manganese, lead, mercury, selenium, silver, and zinc.[60]

**Artichoke (Cynara scolymus)**: Extremely safe, well-studied nutrient that has antioxidant, choleretic, hepatoprotective, bile-enhancing and lipid-lowering effects.[61 62 63 64 65]

## *Directions*

1-2 capsules can be taken three times per day preferably 30 minutes away from food.

Find **AI** on our store at
**shop.ConnersClinic.com/ai**

---


[60] Boyer JL. Bile formation and secretion. Compr Physiol. 2013;3(3):1035"1078. doi:10.1002/cphy.c120027

[61] Salem, B et al Pharmacological Studies of Artichoke Leaf Extract and Their Health Benefits. Plant Foods Hum Nutr. 2015 Dec;70(4):441-53. doi: 10.1007/s11130-015-0503-8

[62] Kirchhoff, R. et al. Increase in choleresis by means of artichoke extract. Results of a randomized placebo-controlled double-blind study. Phytomed- icine 1994; 1: 107

[63] Held C. Artischoke bei Gallenwegsdyskinesien: Workshop â€œNeue Aspekte zur Therapie mit Chloretika. Kluvensiek. 1991; 2:9. Cited in Kraft K. Artichoke leaf extractâ€"Recent findings reflecting effects on lipid metabolism, liver and gastrointestinal tracts. Phytomedicine. 1997; 4(4):369-378

[64] Rondanelli M. et al Health-promoting properties of artichoke in preventing cardiovascular disease by its lipidic and glycemic-reducing action. Monaldi Arch Chest Dis. 2013 Mar;80(1):17-26

[65] El-Boshy M1et al Studies on the protective effect of the artichoke (Cynara scolymus) leaf extract against cadmium toxicity-induced oxidative stress, hepatorenal damage, and immunosuppressive and hematological disorders in rats. Environ Sci Pollut Res Int. 2017 May;24(13):12372-12383

# Other Therapies to Consider for Phase 2 & 3

## Genetic Testing

Each person has a set of genes - about 20,000 in all. The differences between people come from slight variations in these genes. For example, a person with red hair doesn't have the "red hair gene" while a person with brown hair does has the "brown hair gene." Instead, all people have genes for hair color, and different versions of these genes dictate whether someone will be a redhead or a brunette.

Your body contains 50 trillion cells, and almost every one of them contains the complete set of instructions for making you. These instructions are encoded in your DNA.

To make new cells, an existing cell divides in two. But first it copies its DNA so the new cells will each have a complete set of genetic instructions. For a multitude of reasons, cells sometimes make mistakes during the copying process - kind of like typos. These typos lead to variations in the DNA sequence at particular locations, called single nucleotide polymorphisms, or SNPs (pronounced "snips".)

SNPs can generate biological variation between people by causing differences in the recipes for proteins that are written in genes. Those differences can in turn influence a variety of traits such as appearance, disease susceptibility, response to drugs, ability to detoxify quickly or slowly, ability to heal, kill pathogens, and even increase your risk of cancer.

Looking at genetic SNP tests help us shape your specific treatment protocol to best aide your ability to recover from disease. While we "never treat the SNP", we may utilize the information to better treat *you*.

Genetic testing for those with Lyme is *very important*. It can tell us an enormous amount of data that can help us better manage their case. Honestly, I recommend genetic testing for *every* patient I consult with.

Lyme patients in particular need to know if they have SNP defects in their cytochrome P450, SOD, and Glutathione pathways. For example, SOD SNPs leave excess superoxide ions in tissues that bind to a chemical called cytokine-inducible nitric oxide that is in abundance in Chronic Lyme patients. This forms a highly reactive and dangerous compound called peroxynitrate that can actually be the *cause* of many of the symptoms Phase 2 & 3 Lyme patients suffer from!
See the videos on our website at
**ConnersClinic.com/genetic-snp-testing**

# Rife Technology (Energy Medicine)

Many of our Lyme patients start with only using the Rife machine. We **highly** recommend that you seek professional advice when using the Rife and getting it programmed for your needs.

It's *very important* that everyone starts **very slowly** when using the Rife as *it works effectively* and can kill quite quickly, causing Herx reactions. **Do not** get aggressive in your hope to get rid of your disease as fast as possible. **Go slow**!

All cells are capable of receiving a countless number of frequencies that are stored within the cytoplasm of each cell, which itself, consists of H2O. Hydrogen and Oxygen hold the electromagnetic charges, and the cellular memory is then processed within the DNA of each cell. Vital life energy (Bio-energy) fills every cell within the human body, which controls all metabolic processes, including biochemical changes that occur within the cells. It controls the utilization of nutritional substances, and the functioning of all body systems including the immune system.

We predicate that during periods of stress, be it physical or mental stress, this increases the cell's state of vulnerability to discordant frequencies (stressors). For example, electromagnetic fields such as mobile phones, microwaves, computers, household wiring etc. can enter cells through the

Integral membrane proteins in the cell membrane and store in the cytoplasm, altering the cell's homeostasis. Cells are most vulnerable during periods of stress: the greater the stress, the greater the incidence of acquiring homeostatic imbalance.

By recognizing discordant frequencies within cells, the body is more capable of achieving homeostasis. Every disease state and pathogen has its associated harmonic and disharmonic frequencies. Generally speaking, harmonic frequencies maintain health (homeostasis) and promote growth and healing, while disharmonic frequencies produce illness and death (homeostatic imbalance.)


## Everything is Energy

*"The cell is a machine driven by energy. It can thus be approached by studying matter, or by studying energy. In every culture and in every medical tradition before ours, healing was accomplished by moving energy."*
*-Albert Szent-Gyorgyi, Nobel Laureate in Medicine*

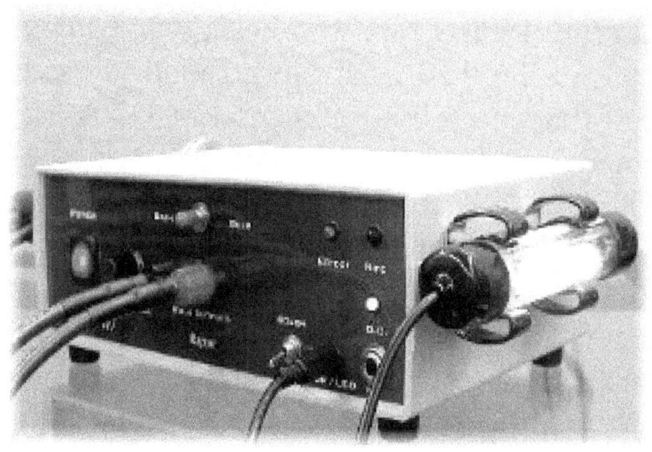

We only suggest using the TrueRife brand of Rife equipment. Most of our cancer and Chronic Lyme patients go home with this machine that we personally program for the patient.

New research introduces a radical understanding of cell science. New biology concepts reveal that human beings control their genome rather than being controlled by it. It is now recognized that environmental frequencies and more specifically, our perception or interpretation of the environment, directly controls the activity of our genes.

This new paradigm of "bio-electrical interaction" has given us a better understanding of how the human body uses energy to heal itself and regulate its activities. It has also enabled science to reevaluate previously discarded medical therapies and to explore new ones based on this interaction.

During the 1990s, three Nobel Prize winners in medicine in the field of advanced medical research revealed that the primary function of DNA lies not in protein synthesis, as widely believed, but in electromagnetic energy reception and transmission. Less than three percent of DNA's function is in protein formulation; more than ninety percent of the DNA functions in the realm of bioelectric signaling. You might say that electromagnetism is fundamentally responsible for all life, and everything in the physical universe. It is also in the spiritual force or energy that gives rise to all matter.[66]

## Other Supplements, Therapies, and Technology

We utilize several other therapies available to local patients, including:

**Hyperthermia** – FIR hyperthermia is Japanese technology utilized also in the Mexican and German cancer clinics

**Neurofeedback** – NFB can help balance brain activity and reduce inflammation, bring clarity,

---

[66] Bioelectromagnetic Healing, its History and a Rationale for its Use Thomas F. Valone, Integrity Research Institute, 1220 L Street NW, Suite 100-232 Washington DC 20005, www.IntegrityResearchInstitute.org Proceedings of the Whole Person Healing Conference, Bethesda, MD, 2003

balance neurotransmitters, reduce brain fog, improve memory, and improve overall function

**Pulsed Electromagnetic Frequency** – PEMF is a tool to bring back cell voltage and improve cell membrane health

**Homeopathy** – The use of different Lyme Borellia and co-infection homeopaths have proven to be highly effective for many of our patients. While some people in Phase 3 may react negatively to homeopaths, most do well if they slowly increase the dose. We recommend titrating up the dosing, starting very slow.

**Other Th2 Stimulants** – As noted earlier in this book, you can dose different nutrients individually as long as they are not known immune (Th1) stimulants. While we believe that everyone is an individual and can react very differently to supplementation, the best remedy may be starting at minimal doses.

**Pulsing Supplements** – We have also found that sensitive patients may benefit from pulsing their supplementation. This means that you would not necessarily take them every day. You may choose to start as slowly as once per week and titrate up from

135

there. I hope you are getting the idea that, in many cases, less is more and slow is better.

Specific, personalized testing that goes far beyond this book

To learn more about Rife technology and other therapies we utilize, visit **ConnersClinic.com**